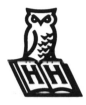

Also by Joseph Juliano

The Diabetic's Innovative Cookbook:
A Positive Approach to Living with Diabetes,
with Dianne Young, Henry Holt, 1994

When Diabetes Complicates Your Life:
Meeting the Challenge and Related Complications
Head-On, Chronimed, 1992

The

DIABETIC MALE'S
ESSENTIAL GUIDE
TO LIVING WELL

❖ ❖ ❖

Joseph Juliano, M.D.

Henry Holt and Company | New York

Henry Holt and Company, Inc.
Publishers since 1866
115 West 18th Street
New York, New York 10011

Henry Holt® is a registered
trademark of Henry Holt and Company, Inc.

Library of Congress Cataloging-in-Publication Data
Juliano, Joseph.
The diabetic male's essential guide to living well /
Joseph Juliano.
p.   cm.
Includes bibliographical references and index.
ISBN 0-8050-3883-3 (hardcover: alk. paper)
1. Diabetes—Popular works.   2. Men—Diseases.
3. Men—Health and hygiene.   I. Title.
RC660.4.J849   1998   97-20310
616.4'62'081—dc21

Henry Holt books are available for special promotions and
premiums. For details contact: Director, Special Markets.

First Edition 1998

Designed by Victoria Hartman

Printed in the United States of America
All first editions are printed on acid-free paper. ∞

2   4   6   8   10   9   7   5   3   1

I dedicate this book to F. J. Weishuhn, M.D., my lifelong family practitioner, who in March 1986 came to my house in the early hours of a Sunday morning, pumped sixty grams of intravenous glucose into me, and saved me from a near-death hypoglycemic coma, and to Max Ellenberg, M.D., and Harold Rifkin, M.D., my mentors in endocrinology and diabetology.

Contents

Acknowledgments

I would like to give special thanks for their help to Stacy Bell, M.D., Harvard Medical School, Medical Foods, Inc., Boston, Massachusetts; James D. Brosseau, M.D., Endocrinology, Grand Forks, North Dakota; Ed Bryant, Diabetes Action Network of the National Federation of the Blind, Columbia, Missouri; Charles E. Ebel, D.D.S., Dentistry, La Grange, Texas; Janice Friday, M.D., Internal Medicine, Smithville, Texas; Kenneth A. Goldberg, M.D., Urology, Male Health Institute, Dallas, Texas; Jo Ann Hoffman, Osbon Medical Systems, Augusta, Georgia; Lee Laris, M.D., Dermatology, Medical Hair Restoration, Phoenix, Arizona; Matt Leavitt, M.D., Executive Director, Medical Hair Restoration, Maitland, Florida; Helen Maidment, M.D. Nephrology, Austin Diagnostic Clinic, Austin, Texas; Dorothy Peterson, R.N., The Geddings Osbon Medical Foundation Impotence Resource Center, Augusta, Georgia; John Raia, Pharm. D., Bristol-Myers Squibb Pharmaceuticals, Plainsboro, New Jersey; Vladimir Rizov, M.D., Conservative Therapy Clinic, Austin, Texas; Ron Scott, M.D., Wound Care Clinic of North Texas, Dallas, Texas; Jeff Tsing, M.D., Master Acupuncturist, Texas College of Traditional Chinese Medicine, Austin, Texas; Richard Wiesner, World-Wide President, LifeScan, Inc., a Johnson and Johnson Company, Milpitas, California; Jeff Zwiefel, Exercise Physiology, NordicTrack, Minneapolis, Minnesota.

My thanks go also to Beth Crossman, my editor at Henry Holt who, under the most trying situations, has again encouraged me to improve my writing and help me to produce what I truly believe is a good book, and to Vicki Underwood, Ph.D., who spent countless hours editing a difficult manuscript.

• • •

The following people helped me in many ways to write this book and I thank them all: Vic Juliano, Jo Ann Juliano, Patricia Elaine Addison, Michael Donahue, Bobby Macpherson, Hank Belopavlovich, Rise Ciufia, Randy Kay, Jim Lloyd, Pat Haley, Betty Taylor, Johnny Pittman, Dr. Ann Yakimovicz, Ellen Stuart, Monte Stuart, Rick Womack, Jill Kendrick, Cheri Andrews, Monica Wofford, Laurie Wyeth, Alba Chronis, Gena Chronis, Clyde Stech, Leslie Taylor, Dr. John Carey, Linda Shirocky, Sylvia Thoung, Joy Robinson, Charlie Claiborne, Mary Claiborne, and Rosemary Merritt.

Foreword

For many years, Hank Belopavlovich was a senior lecturer for the Silva Method of Self Mind Control, a system developed over twenty-five years ago by José Silva to utilize the mind by engaging the right brain, the intuitive side of the brain, in order to set in motion visual imagery to heal oneself and make life better through positive thought processes.

Hank does not have diabetes himself, but he has taught the course to hundreds of people and has worked with many diabetics. He has introduced me to several disciplines of positive self mind control, areas I have successfully used to improve my life with diabetes and blindness.

Here is what he says about positive attitudinal healing and using the mind to create a positive self-image and healthy body.

How can we regulate our lives? Of primary importance is to be in control. What happens when things beyond our control affect us? Do we react or respond?

What works for me may not work for you, or what works for me just may work for you. This is all added to our perception, our action, or our reaction to any given situation. This process is what we call our life experience.

Life is an experience and we are cocreators of this experience. We can be conscious or oblivious to it, and each one of us has the opportunity to do something about it if we so desire.

Where do we begin? Know thyself, control thyself. It sounds easy enough and has been known for centuries, but what does it mean and can we accomplish this? A set of tools is needed. They come in different varieties and are applied in different ways. The tools we are speaking about are mind tools and are just as particular to the mind as a set of socket wrenches are to an engine block. These tools are applied to harness the potential to work on the engine block that sits on our shoulders. Realize that it is your brain and mind that govern your body. They run and regulate everything from your blood, to individual cell replacement, to nutrient distribution. It is a master biochemical computer in control of a massive biological system.

What are we to do when we find that we are our own worst enemies, primarily because of our beliefs developed over a lifetime and our level of consciousness and awareness? Is to know thyself and control thyself poppycock or fact? Reading this book is a start. Opening up the mind empowers the opening of doors to knowledge gained from within it. It requires hard work to "work" on ourselves, and we have different aspects on which to work, depending upon specific conditions.

Our health is also determined by our diets, as we are what we eat physically and mentally. What foodstuffs do you run your motor on? It is important to eat healthy, clean food, including more fruits and vegetables, with an eye always toward balance. Convert to organically grown fruits and vegetables if you can, as a vitally important part of your diet. Include grains and cereals while avoiding processed sugars.

How do you feed your brain mentally? We consume the environment around us, which conditions our attitudes. Our work, our homes, and all the people around us influence the mental diet. Even the television programs we watch greatly influence our mental state. Where do we find organically grown mental food? We must grow our own. It is important to understand that mind guides brain, which in turn guides the body. How do we do this? A recipe is required that is suitable to our individual taste. Several recommendations include the martial arts, karate being one of the best for mind-body coordination, and another is developing a program of self mind control. Disciplining the mind and working with it gives us control over the body. The object is to stop the terrible complications of diabetes, or, at the least, do the best job we can to manage it.

How important is this work? Your length and quality of life depend on it. When you are asked to change or modify your lifestyle, you will need inner strength to carry it through. You will be put to the test. These recommendations are ways to prepare and do what it takes to make it happen. It is nothing fancy; just plain work and honest effort to help oneself are all that's required. This self knowledge is crucial to the existence on this planet, whether or not you have a particular malady. Because you do have diabetes, this mental power becomes a survival tool. It will allow you to realize and utilize your inner resources and apply them consciously to a particular problem at hand. What more could we ask for? Free will is at hand, so go to work.

—HANK BELOPAVLOVICH

Introduction

I am a car fanatic. In my opinion, the finest sports car in the world is the Ferrari Testa Rossa 512 M. The engine is an engineering masterpiece with its classic V-12 configuration, four cams, forty-eight valves, and silky smooth computerized electronic fuel injection. The noise from the precision gearing and melding of engine parts, along with a computerized tuned exhaust, is like a symphony tuning up in all its glory. This Ferrari is an incredibly sexy-looking machine with a hand-detailed aluminum body by the famous coachworks of Pininfarina in Italy. The engine parts are built by automotive craftsmen with the finest machine tools in the world. The finest leather is used for the interior, along with beautifully detailed Italian Veglia instruments. The slotted gearbox looks like it came from a Ferrari Formula One racing car, which it did. The alloy wheels are balanced to within a tenth of a gram of each other for sustained speeds of over 180 miles per hour.

Now ask yourself a question: Do you want your body to be like a Ferrari, sleek, fast, and in the finest tune, or do you want it to be like a tired sedan, just barely running enough to prevent itself from falling apart at all corners?

As a diabetic male, I prefer to think of my body as a Ferrari. That's right, guys, a Ferrari costs more to maintain and keep running properly, and thus is a lot more work and effort than some cheap pile of junk, but, come on, wouldn't you really rather be driving the best?

So, if you are a car fanatic like I am, using only the finest fuel, oil, waxes, and finish preservers, then why should we not treat our wonderful male human bodies, that just happen to have this medical condition we call diabetes, as well as we would the finest automobile in the world? I suppose we take our bodies for granted at times, especially when we're young.

Certainly, when I was first diagnosed with insulin-dependent diabetes over thirty years ago at age fifteen, I was a long way from the understanding of how the aging process and the concomitant progressive nature of diabetes mellitus would influence my life forever. If you are a newly diagnosed male diabetic, you will face many challenges in determining the changes in lifestyle encountered in dealing with diabetes, whether it is insulin-dependent or non-insulin-dependent diabetes.

As you come to terms with your diagnosis, you need to become a medical expert about the condition you must deal with on a daily basis. Read as much as you can in the diabetes journals, and study as many books as you can get your hands on, in order to understand this disease in the broadest terms. I have tried my best to supply you with copious references and resource materials in this book. However, there are many more available than are listed here. Remember, this book is not intended as a self-management resource in toto; rather it is a source for managing issues faced by the male diabetic population.

Because as diabetics we must pay closer attention to the care and fine-tuning aspects of our bodies, as we discussed with the Ferrari example, we must work harder, more intelligently, more diligently, and with even greater discipline than nondiabetics. I have determined that this is entirely right for me and I am challenged every day to improve my health by exercising more, watching my diet even more closely, and paying meticulous attention to my insulin therapy.

There are other issues we face as males and as male diabetics, and it is these very issues that provided me with the inspiration to write this book and undergo the various health techniques discussed herein. I feel very strongly that if I discuss a particular health technique, then I should at least try the technique on myself. Because I have had diabetes for thirty years, and have been totally blind due to complications of diabetic retinopathy for ten years now, I consider myself a gold standard in determining health techniques that would be advantageous to my better health.

For example, I continue with acupuncture treatments today. Do I think you should jump into acupuncture treatments for yourself?

Certainly not, unless you thoroughly discuss this subject with your doctor, study the chapter I have written in this book, and consider what acupuncture has done for a long-term diabetic such as myself. What about male-pattern baldness and diabetes? If you are a young man, this subject may be the furthest thing from your mind. However, a brief study of today's modern techniques will better prepare you for the future, should this become a concern. Obviously, this same reasoning can be applied to the subject of diabetic male impotence. This is one area of health for men that can cause great anxiety, emotional and psychological tension, stress, and, if left unchecked, a great deal of depression. So let's discuss it, study it, and become familiar with this process as a potential complication in the life of a diabetic male.

In the first part of this book, we will discuss long-term complications that may occur with diabetes. This should not be considered a fatalistic approach to dealing with diabetes in the long term, but rather an educational opportunity to better understand and deal with the ramifications that may or may not be a part of your life with diabetes. Knowledge represents power and strength. The more you know about this disease, the more powerful you will be in dealing with it on a daily basis. Please understand that this book is not a textbook or a scientific treatise on the male diabetic, but a resource for further study to be used in conjunction with discussions with your own physician.

You will find that I continually stress the vital importance of several key elements. First and foremost, it is imperative that you discuss all aspects of your diabetes with your own personal health care team. This team usually consists of a general practitioner or internal medicine specialist, an endocrinologist who is a specialist in the treatment of diabetes, a nurse practitioner, and a registered dietician.

Second, good management of your diabetes is imperative.

Third, if you are a Type I insulin-dependent diabetic, blood glucose testing is a requirement and a natural part of your diabetic management regime, as natural as your insulin dose. If you are an insulin-dependent diabetic, you must check your blood glucose every day; this means two to six finger prick blood tests per day.

Fourth and finally, if you have diabetes, insulin-dependent or not, do not smoke. If you smoke at this time, please get help and quit immediately. If you are a young man or teenager with diabetes, remember what a very wise vascular surgeon professor once said: If you have diabetes, you can choose between your cigarettes or your legs, but you can't have both.

As we become accustomed to the daily routine of diabetes, we may be tempted to take certain liberties and shortcuts. I know this because it certainly happened to me. Try your best not to let a lackadaisical attitude destroy your respect for the exceedingly complex nature of diabetes. Keep in mind that diabetes can sneak up on you. Ultimately, although I would like you to be challenged and inspired by all that I am telling you, I am taking the risk that you will interpret my pieces of advice as grave warnings, admonitions, predictions of defeat, and misery. "What the hell," you may say, "it's going to happen to me anyway, so why should I take good care of my diabetes?" I fully understand this attitude. However, we must always keep the goal in mind of good diabetes maintenance. Diabetes is an insidious disease. It allows you many liberties for an unspecified amount of time; then, seemingly all at once, the whole world falls in on you as the years add complications.

Now, let's prepare to enter into the improved health care techniques and issues that are of interest to the male diabetic. Open your mind, but always remember that good common sense and logic along with good standard medical practice are the watchwords of everything that is written here.

I wish you the best of luck in dealing with your own case of diabetes.

Take a Walk with Me

O what a lonely journey
Perennial darkness can be,
But, perchance, an Angel from Heaven
Has chosen to accompany me.

O loneliness, O torturous void,
Sans the Almighty, I have cried out
In disdain and despair.

O praise the Almighty, you have both come to me
In spiritual reunification.

I walk alone with an Angel from Heaven.
Her thoughts comfort me,
and mine, her.
I am with her every waking hour
As her spirit and soul touch me and remind me
      I am with her.

The darkened path has taken on renewed light,
The loneliness given way to sweet kindness
      and companionship.

Take a walk with me,
My sweet Angel from Heaven.
As I heal you will heal,
As I achieve, you will achieve.

As I walk this life alone,
I will not be alone.

You are with me, my Angel.

Take a walk with me.

Joseph Juliano
April 1997

DIABETIC MALE'S ESSENTIAL GUIDE TO LIVING WELL

✧ ✧ ✧

1

Gaining a Perspective
on Diabetes

Okay, let's go for it. We will examine the differences between Type I and Type II diabetes mellitus and then explore the history of this very ancient disease. We will briefly look at the role insulin plays for the insulin-dependent diabetic and at the different types of insulin used in today's modern therapy. Then, we will plunge into a study of oral antidiabetic agents used to control the blood sugar of a non-insulin-dependent diabetic. A clear understanding will be gained as to why a Type I diabetic cannot take pills to control his diabetes and why a Type II diabetic may not have to take pills at all, or may have to take pills and insulin injections together.

A General Discussion of Diabetes Mellitus,
Type I and Type II

In 1979 the National Diabetes Data Group, NDDG, part of the National Institutes of Health, determined a new classification of diabetes and other categories of glucose intolerance. If you are insulin-dependent, and therefore must administer your daily insulin dose or doses with a syringe or other insulin delivery device, then you have what is referred to as Type I insulin-dependent diabetes mellitus, IDDM. At one time this type of diabetes was referred to as juvenile-onset diabetes or simply juvenile diabetes. This type of diabetes encompasses about 20 percent of all diabetic cases. It is characterized by severe reduction of available insulin in children and young adults. In these cases overt symptoms are present, including polyuria (frequent urination), polydipsia (excessive thirst), weight loss, and, many times, ketoacidosis. Diabetic ketoacidosis, DKA, is a serious condition of prolonged high blood sugar, increased acid concentration, and decreased bicarbonate along with an accumulation of ketone bodies (see Chapter 9, page 62).

If you are able to control your diabetes with diet, exercise, and/or oral medication, then you have Type II non-insulin-dependent diabetes mellitus, NIDDM. This type of diabetes was once referred to as adult-onset diabetes. Making up 80 percent of the diabetic population, it is characterized by insulin resistance and usually occurs in patients over the age of forty, with decreased tissue response to their own, endogenous, insulin and/or decreased tissue response to insulin given by injection, an exogenous source.

Onset of Type II diabetes is difficult to determine, and many cases will be asymptomatic for years. Obesity is a problem in 60 to 90 percent of Type II cases. Today, the classifications of Type I and Type II are used so as not to confuse an adult who has been diagnosed with insulin-dependent diabetes. Certainly juvenile-onset diabetes would not be the appropriate designation for this type of diabetes.

There are three key components to managing your diabetes, whether you have Type I or Type II: proper diet, the right amount of exercise, and careful administration of insulin or the oral anti-diabetic agent your doctor has prescribed.

One key point you need to understand very clearly: every single case of diabetes is an individual case and thus represents issues, treatments, and particular challenges that are part of that individual's own genetic makeup. My case of diabetes will be different from yours, and although there may be broad generalizations we can make concerning my diabetes and yours, there will be many differences. Because of this fact, it is imperative that you discuss your case of diabetes with your doctor on a regular basis, to allow him or her to become familiar with your own individual case.

If you have been diagnosed with Type II non-insulin-dependent diabetes, you may find it intriguing that some individuals who have been formally diagnosed with this type of diabetes have been able to regulate their diets so carefully that they no longer have diabetes. A dear friend of mine, Don, was diagnosed with Type II diabetes several years ago, when he was in his mid-fifties. After the initial shock and consequent depression, my extremely disciplined friend did a complete lifestyle about-face when he found he was diabetic. At six feet two inches tall and 190 pounds, cholesterol at 350 mg/dl, triglycerides (blood fats) at 400 plus, he lost fifty pounds and reduced his cholesterol and triglycerides to near-normal levels. He dieted himself out of diabetes and greatly improved his health. The end result of his extremely disciplined dieting was that he lost fifty pounds, yet he was not overweight to begin with. He looked like he was only skin and bones, but more important to him was that he did not have to take any oral medication for his diabetes because his blood sugars were and are now running at normal levels. Some mutual friends and I had a rather frank talk with him and we told him it was time to increase his caloric intake on his diabetic diet so that he would not dry up and blow away. He took our advice and gained some weight and is in great shape today. The moral of this story is that it can be done no matter what, understanding that real dedication and discipline in confronting the challenge of diabetes can result in making the entire process easier to live with and manage.

Diabetes from a Historical Perspective

Let us define diabetes mellitus. Literally translated, mellitus means honey (or sugar), and diabetes means siphon (or tube). When translated freely, diabetes mellitus means a running through of sugar, which certainly describes the condition in its uncontrolled state.

Maturity-onset or adult-onset Type II diabetes mellitus is defined as an often milder form of diabetes of gradual onset in obese individuals over the age of thirty-five. These definitions cover the term *diabetes* in the broadest sense.

Diabetes is a disease going back to ancient times, believed to date to at least 1550 B.C., due to the mention of the term *polyuria* in the ancient writings of the Egyptian Ebers Papyrus. Frequent urination is indeed a symptom of diabetes, and thus medical historians believe that this is the first mention of the disease in recorded history. There are medical writings from India that may precede the Egyptian writings. In these ancient writings, it was noted that honey was present in the urine of some people, and other symptoms of diabetes were reported, including thirst, fatigue, and skin eruptions. These writings from India also proclaimed that this disease was found among the wealthy and immoderate. In this context, immoderate most probably denotes those who ate and drank too much. Additionally, some possibilities of hereditary effects of this disorder were noted during this time. Physicians proclaimed this disease incurable. Other medical writings from this same period include the Chinese, who reported polyuria and the sweet taste of an affected person's urine that would attract dogs. Persons affected were also found to possess the skin eruptions or boils reported in other ancient writings.

However, in the medical writings of the ancient Greeks, most notably Hippocrates, there is no mention of diabetes. This is thought to be due to the fact that the ancient Greeks lived severe and austere lives with little obsessive consumption. As time moved forward and the lifestyle improved for the Greeks, excessive behavior (excessive in this context meaning eating and drinking too much) became evident in their writings of a kidney disease known to them as diarrhea of the urine. Medical historians believe this to be an early description of another symptom of diabetes.

In the fourth century Arab physicians reported honey in the urine, and during the Renaissance physicians reported that diabetics drank less than they excreted; they were amazed at the tremendous quantity of urine diabetics produced. During the sixteenth and seventeenth centuries in England, more knowledge was gained concerning diabetes and an important finding was made that sweetness in the urine was determined to be caused by the presence of sugar.

In the nineteenth century the German physician, Johann Franz, developed a yeast test to determine the presence of sugar in the urine. Up until this time, the only way to detect the presence of sugar in a suspected diabetic's urine was to taste it.

Diabetes has been suspected to be a disease of the stomach, the kidneys, the liver, and the blood. It was thought to be a central nervous system disease until about 1857. Minkowski and von Mering conducted experiments in 1889 in Strassburg, Germany, to prove that diabetes is a disease associated with the pancreas. This was an important finding and one that is often forgotten in the history of diabetes.

Eugene L. Opie, in 1901, and Leonid Sobelev, in 1902, determined that diabetes is a disease of the endocrine system. Their experiments discovered that a group of special cells in the pancreas were part of the endocrine system. These cells were named the islets of Langerhans after the man who first described these cells, Paul Langerhans, a German anatomist and physician who had discovered them in 1869. These islet cells deposit their hormones directly into the bloodstream. Unfortunately, Langerhans did not have an understanding of the function of the cells that carry his name. It was later discovered by Opie and Sobelev that the hormonal secretions were affected by beta cells whose function was changed, resulting in diabetes. At this point, it was understood that a specific antidiabetic hormone existed, and the investigative race was on to isolate this specific hormone that would be usable in the treatment of diabetes. By isolating the hormone from dog pancreas, two Canadian physicians, Frederick G. Banting and Charles H. Best, discovered insulin in 1921 and later won the Nobel Prize in Physiology and Medicine. According to the *Encyclopedia of Medical History,* "the Nobel Prize committee botched the award. Herbert Best, who worked with Frederick Banting throughout the project's life, received no prize. McLeod [the proprietor of the laboratory where Banting and Best did their research] was named discoverer of insulin despite the fact that he was away throughout the discovery period, and played no part in the actual research of insulin. The vagaries of the prize committee were partially redressed when Banting shared his prize with Best."

2

Insulin

Insulin is a very complex and large protein molecule. It is also a special hormone, which is produced by the pancreas, a gland of internal secretion found in the endocrine system. Insulin is produced by specialized cells called beta cells found within the islets of Langerhans within the pancreas gland. The pancreas serves many more purposes than just to secrete insulin. It is a complex organ with many functions and plays a crucial role in the secretion of digestive enzymes, the chemicals used in the breakdown of food in the metabolic process.

You may well be aware of the importance of insulin in controlling blood sugar, but I would like to mention a few more facts concerning the importance of insulin as it relates to the biochemistry of metabolism. If you want to read further into the molecular biology of diabetes, there are many excellent technical works on the biochemistry of diabetes. In my opinion, the best medical textbook covering this subject is *Diabetes Mellitus Theory and Practice, Third Edition*, edited by Max Ellenberg, M.D., and Harold Rifkin, M.D., and published in 1988 (page 188).

We have seen that insulin is manufactured, stored, secreted, and placed directly into the bloodstream by the beta cells located on the islets of Langerhans. Insulin plays a vital role in metabolism, the myriad complex phenomena associated with the derivation of energy from the acquisition of various materials required to sustain life and promote further growth. Thus, ingested food is broken down into various components through this complex process, known as metabolism. This derived energy is then utilized and stored to sustain vital functions. The metabolic process continues even though there may be no ingestion of food as the complex biochemical interactions continue in order to make and repair cells and tissues. Without insulin, a vital component to the metabolic process is missing, thus causing a negative domino effect to occur during metabolism. Because the human body is an absolute miracle in its ability to biochemically interplay one process with another, insulin plays an important role in augmenting certain processes that remove sugar from the blood and inhibiting other processes that act to raise the blood sugar.

An example of the stimulatory effect of insulin is its effect on the liver to make and store an important animal starch called glycogen. Insulin is also the necessary regulatory hormone in the process by which sugar is removed from the blood and allowed to enter into muscle and fat cells. These few examples are part of insulin's ability to lower the blood sugar and thus keep homeostasis, or the normal balanced condition within the body. As insulin augments and stimulates, conversely insulin is an inhibitory substance also. It inhibits the breakdown of glycogen within the liver by inhibiting the process of glycogenolysis (breakdown of animal starch), which would turn animal starch back into sugar. Another important role of insulin is the inhibition of new sugar formation, or gluconeogenesis, from within the liver. By inhibiting these two processes, insulin lowers the blood sugar via alternative pathways.

Insulin also plays a vital role in causing the entrance of sugar, and thus energy, into fat and protein cells. Without insulin, amino acids, the body's basic building blocks, would not be stimulated into delivery to the muscle cells, and thus would not promote the buildup of muscle tissue.

Without insulin, the above important pathways would not happen. Thus the uncontrolled diabetic, or the diabetic in need of insulin therapy, tends to deteriorate due to the lack of these important cell- and tissue-building pathways. This is a very basic overview of insulin and its affect on biochemical pathways. Its action within the human body is crucial to our understanding of the human condition.

Types of Insulin

There are four basic categories of insulin defined by its onset and duration. The onset refers to the time the insulin takes to begin exerting its effect. The duration refers to the total time of action in terms of its effect.

Super-quick-acting Insulin

Eli Lilly's new super-quick-acting insulin is, at the present time, in a class by itself. This insulin begins its action within fifteen minutes after injection and peaks in one hour. This insulin is for high blood sugar situations where immediate control is necessary. For now, this insulin is available only with your doctor's prescription, and consultation with your doctor is mandatory before using this new insulin preparation.

Short-acting Insulin

Short-acting insulin, usually referred to as regular insulin, or Humulin R, has an onset of between twenty and thirty minutes. Its action will peak, that is, deliver its highest level of performance, in three to five hours. Its duration, or its total time of effect, is from five to seven hours. This insulin type is clear and requires no rolling action to insure its proper mixing within the vial. Regular insulin has been traditionally used in conjunction with other insulin types. Today, a new therapy is to use regular insulin alone, but in four to six injections spread throughout a twenty-four-hour period.

Intermediate-acting Insulin

Intermediate-acting insulin, called N when composed of human insulin or NPH or Lente when it is a mixture of pork and beef insulin, has an onset of sixty to ninety minutes. The peak action of intermediate-acting insulin is from eight to twelve hours. The duration of this insulin is from twenty-four to forty-eight hours. This insulin type is cloudy and must be carefully rolled in the palms of the hands to insure good mixing. Never shake this type of insulin to mix it. Insulin is a delicate protein and should never be vigorously agitated. Shaking also will produce frothing or bubbles, which will make it more difficult to withdraw.

Long-acting Insulin

Long-acting insulin, known as Ultralente, has an onset of five to eight hours. This insulin peaks in sixteen to eighteen hours, while the duration is thirty-two or more hours. Ultralente supplies a basal level of insulin and must be used with multiple doses of regular insulin. This insulin is also cloudy in appearance and should always be carefully rolled in the palms of the hands to insure proper mixing, just as in the case of intermediate-acting insulin.

First introduced by a pharmaceutical company in Denmark, single-vial preparation of premixed insulin is now available composed of NPH intermediate-acting insulin and regular insulin in a two-to-one ratio. That is, the ratio of the two components of insulin is two parts of NPH intermediate-acting insulin to one part of regular, short-acting insulin. If you were to take thirty units of this insulin, using the two-to-one ratio, you would be taking ten units of regular insulin with twenty units of NPH intermediate-acting insulin, for a total dose of thirty units. I would carefully evaluate the convenience of the single-vial approach against the additional versatility of mixing regular and NPH insulin using two separate vials. The Danish preparation is difficult for the beginner to maneuver, and even for the veteran diabetic it can be a very complicated insulin to use. By all means check with your doctor and be sure you understand this insulin well before you and your doctor agree that it is the correct insulin for your needs. It is a cloudy-appearing insulin due to the presence of NPH intermediate-acting insulin. The same care in mixing before use is indicated as in the case of the other cloudy-appearing insulins. Remember that regular insulin is always clear in the vial. If it looks slightly cloudy, it must be discarded.

How does a blind person know which insulin is which? Learn by feel, and carefully examine the shapes of the various vials of insulins. The vial of regular insulin, if manufactured in Denmark by Nordisk, was once shaped differently than the vial of N or NPH. This greatly helped in identifying the insulin type, and making sure one was taking the right amount. Unfortunately, at this time Eli Lilly is not differentiating its regular vials of insulin from its NPH or other insulins. The Diabetics' Division of the National Federation of the Blind has undertaken the tremendously huge task of trying to convince the Federal Food and Drug Administration and Eli Lilly, the largest manufacturer of insulin in the world, to manufacture their vials with different shapes so as not to confuse either the sighted or the blind diabetic population. We are all anxiously awaiting new FDA and corporate guidelines to address this very important issue within the diabetic world. Eli Lilly has informed the National Federation of the Blind and other consumer groups that it has some promising new designs on the drawing board, but due to involvement of new patents, it is not able to divulge its ideas at this time. Eli Lilly predicts there eventually will be a new product available to help diabetics distinguish the different types of insulins. This is great news, and perhaps by the time you read this book, Eli Lilly will have presented its new vial design to the world.

If your normal daily dose is ten units of regular insulin and twenty units of Humulin N insulin, for a total dose of thirty units, and if, for some reason, you are distracted or lose concentration and take twenty units of regular and ten units of Humulin N, an incorrect amount from your normal daily dose, you are in big trouble. The large dose of regular, short-acting insulin will send you into an insulin reaction in less than one hour unless your blood sugar is extremely high. The point here is to always be very careful in your insulin administration and to always double-check yourself. One of the first blind diabetics I met after I lost my eyesight was thirteen years younger than I and had been blind due to diabetic retinopathy for seven years. He was fiercely independent, lived and traveled by himself, and totally managed his diabetes himself. He went to his pharmacist one evening to purchase his insulin, which consisted of mixing regular insulin with a larger dose of NPH intermediate-acting insulin. Instead of giving him his usual insulin prescription, the pharmacist mistakenly gave him two vials of regular insulin. The next morning, this diabetic mixed his insulins, which consisted of twelve units of regular and forty units of NPH, or so he thought. What he actually took was fifty-two units of regular, fast-acting insulin. Almost immediately he began feeling the effects of a very serious insulin reaction. He frantically called upon his sighted neighbor in the apartment next door, who had fortunately not yet left for work. The neighbor confirmed this diabetic's worst fear that something was terribly wrong. With presence of mind, this diabetic calmly called 911 and told them to bring intravenous glucose as soon as possible. The neighbor was pouring orange juice into this diabetic as fast as he could, but the effect of this tremendous overdose of regular insulin was taking its toll. Fortunately, the story ended well, with the diabetic receiving enough

IV glucose to sustain his life. Had he waited much longer, this story may have ended tragically.

. . .

Even a veteran diabetic like myself with over thirty-two years of insulin administration has made this error on occasion. Through the years I have made almost every mistake in the book, and I will try to point out these mistakes to indicate the pitfalls that I hope you can avoid.

Generally, the insulin injection time is thirty minutes before meals. When you inject your insulin at this time, it allows an onset interval to elapse before the insulin can take action. This will coincide with the ingestion of your meal, thus making the injection of your insulin as close to the normal pancreas function as possible.

Over the many years since Banting and Best discovered insulin, techniques have vastly improved in insulin's purification process. In the early days, insulin was obtained from the pancreas of cows and pigs since there was a plentiful supply, but the purification processes utilized in order to distribute the life-sustaining fluid were crude at best. I have been told by diabetics with more than fifty years of insulin-dependent diabetes that the early insulin preparations were brown in color due to the blood from the animals from which the insulin had been derived. In modern times, insulin is sometimes still obtained from these sources, but purification techniques have been improved and most insulin produced today is synthetically produced human insulin.

With the introduction of modern genetic engineering and biotechnology, human insulin has been synthesized using the *E. coli* bacteria. The new era of human insulin, that is, insulin that is exactly the same as that found in the human body, amino acid for amino acid, has provided the insulin-dependent diabetic population with a greatly improved insulin source.

The major advantage of human insulin over beef and pork insulins is the absence of allergic irritation or allergic reactions at the injection site. Beef and pork insulins are also prone to cause an insulin-resistance response that can lead to problems in the diabetic patient. Pure pork insulin causes fewer allergic reactions than other nonhuman insulin preparations because it differs only slightly from human insulin. Also, it can be converted to human insulin, giving us another valuable source of human insulin. The cost of pure pork insulin is greater than beef or pork mixtures and may require dose changes. Any change in insulin types requires consultation with your doctor and careful monitoring of your blood sugar. Human insulin provides a match to the naturally occurring human insulin, is very pure, and is not prone to cause allergic reactions and insulin resistance. All this is good evidence, indeed, for you to be using today's modern human insulin.

3

Oral Antidiabetic Medications

According to the American Diabetes Association and other health professionals who care for diabetics, the best treatment for Type II non-insulin-dependent diabetes is losing weight, exercise, and careful dieting. If these techniques do not adequately lower blood sugar levels, then the next step is the administration of oral medication. All types of oral medications designed to lower the blood glucose of a Type II diabetic sold in the United States today are not insulin pills, but members of a class of drugs called sulfonylureas. They work to stimulate the pancreas to produce insulin in sufficient amounts to control blood sugar. There is another class of oral antidiabetic drugs called biguanides that have been prescribed in Europe for three decades, which we will discuss shortly.

The Sulfonylureas

There are six sulfonylurea oral agents available in the United States. The following four oral agents have been used for about twenty-five years: (1) chlorpropamide, trade names Diabinese and Glucamide, (2) tolazamide, trade names Ronase and Tolinase, (3) tolbutamide, trade names Orinase and Oramide, and (4) the rarely used acetohexamide, trade name Dymelor.

In 1984, the second generation of sulfonylureas came into use. These medicines are (1) glipizide, trade named Glucotrol and (2) glyburide, trade named DiaBeta, Glynase, and Micronase. These new drugs can be taken in smaller doses than the first-generation drugs.

All of these sulfonylurea drugs have similar effects on blood glucose levels. What is important to understand is that they differ in side effects, in how often they are taken, and in interactions with other drugs.

The University Group Diabetes Project, UGDP, studied the sulfonylurea drug tolbutamide in the 1970s. This study linked use of tolbutamide with increased risk of death due to heart disease, but the study has been criticized by many diabetes experts who believe the experimental protocol was flawed and the results invalid.

Most diabetes experts conclude that a link between tolbutamide and heart disease is a very weak one, if one exists at all. The issue remains unsettled today, although during the early to mid 1970s it was a hotly debated issue. Today, the labeling on all six drugs alerts doctors to the UGDP findings, even though the study found a link with heart disease for only one sulfonylurea.

The Biguanides

Biguanides, another type of oral antidiabetic drug, have been available and used by those with non-insulin-dependent diabetes in Europe since the 1940s. During the 1970s, treatment with biguanides was not allowed in the United States due to inherent problems with their use, such as lactic acidosis. On December 30, 1994, the Food and Drug Administration approved metformin, a new type of biguanide, trade name Glucophage, for clinical use in the United States. Metformin works as well as the sulfonylurea drugs, does not increase levels of very low density lipoprotein (VLDL, the bad cholesterol), and does not lower blood glucose to dangerously hypoglycemic levels, unlike the sulfonylureas.

For millions of Type II diabetics, the risk of hypoglycemia, low blood sugar, is reduced by metformin due to its nonstimulatory effect on the pancreas. An effective treatment for some Type II diabetics is a combination therapy of metformin and a selected sulfonylurea. Because their modes of action are pharmacologically different, a new era in control for the Type II diabetic may be at hand, especially for those who have experienced difficulty in controlling their blood sugar on a sulfonylurea agent, diet, and exercise alone. In England, where it has been in use for many years, one out of four prescriptions for diabetes pills is for metformin.

Many with Type II diabetes begin with the problem of insulin resistance. Interestingly, their pancreas produces enough insulin, but the cells of their bodies do not respond correctly to their insulin, and thus high blood glucose results. For reasons that are not fully understood, the pancreas of the Type II diabetic, sooner or later, will begin producing less and less insulin. Sulfonylureas boost the insulin output of the pancreas, while also stopping the liver from spilling glycogen, stored glucose, into the blood. Thus, metformin's mode of action in lowering blood glucose is to prevent the liver from spilling glycogen into the blood, while the sulfonylureas stimulate the pancreas to produce insulin. Metformin also lowers insulin resistance while retarding the absorption of food as it is digested in the small intestine.

Will you, as a Type II diabetic, be able to take metformin? This question will be answered by your endocrinologist, who will be able to advise you on the possibility of switching to metformin, according to your case of diabetes, diet, exercise program, and level of blood glucose control.

An abundance of data has been collected from other countries to support the fact that metformin may be useful in preventing weight gain in those Type II diabetics who are more than 20 percent over ideal body weight. Patients with Type II diabetes normally take metformin with meals, two or three times a day.

Should sulfonylurea drug therapy fail, metformin can be used as a secondary defensive measure. Unfortunately, the pancreas of a Type II diabetic may fail after some years of experience with the disease. In this type of case, the only step after metformin or a combination therapy using metformin and a sulfonylurea is the use of insulin injections.

As is the case with any drug, metformin does have some side effects. Metformin is contraindicated, that is, should not be prescribed, in patients with heart, kidney, or liver disease. Approximately 20 percent of patients taking metformin complain of gastrointestinal distress after taking the drug. These gastrointestinal problems range from a bitter metallic aftertaste in the mouth to diarrhea. It has been found that these unpleasant side effects tend to diminish after some time on the drug.

From 1959 to 1977, doctors prescribed phenformin (trade named Meltrol, a close relative of metformin) to hundreds of thousands of Type II diabetics. In 1977 the FDA identified over two hundred cases of lactic acidosis in patients who were using this drug and banned the use of phenformin in this country. Lactic acidosis is a very serious condition wherein the blood is poisoned due to a buildup of the acid lactate. As is the case with diabetic ketoacidosis, DKA, lactic acidosis is a difficult biochemical condition to stabilize, which results in shock and even coma, and is fatal in 50 percent of those who develop it. There is some indication that most of the 255 reported cases of lactic acidosis occurred in patients who should not have been treated with metformin, due to accompanying heart, kidney, or liver disease.

4

Self Home Blood
Glucose Monitoring

Self home blood glucose monitoring is one of the most important advances in the field of diabetes since the discovery of insulin in 1922. You have a better chance at closely controlling your diabetes and thus lessening the opportunity for fatal complications by diligently utilizing self home blood glucose monitoring on a daily basis.

There are many things we must do in order to better care for ourselves that are just a real drag. Overall as diabetics, we must live a cleaner, healthier lifestyle. We must undergo adjustments and changes in our diets to better control our diabetes. The ritual of insulin administration, whether it is by syringe, insulin pump, or air jet injection delivery, is, nonetheless, a major component of the diabetic regime. Proper exercise is vitally important and it is a key component to better control and health within the diabetic management regime. Then, of course, there are the myriad details of seeing doctors more regularly, taking adequate precautions against infections, taking proper care of the feet, and management of hypertension, just to name a few.

Self home blood glucose monitoring is something that you must do along with the absolute necessity of never missing your insulin injection, or never forgetting to take your oral medication. Blood glucose monitoring is that important. I know you may be wondering how can it be that lancing your finger, which can sometimes hurt like hell, and obtaining a blood glucose value are as important as the other things we have talked about. What am I supposed to do with these numbers anyway?

The knowledge of the level of blood glucose preceding your insulin injection or a meal is of critical importance to you. For instance, if you are unaware that your blood glucose is precariously low, at around 46 mg/dl, and you take your evening insulin injection, it is paramount that you get food into you right away. At this low level of blood glucose and with your insulin beginning to work for you in thirty minutes or less, you may fall prey to a serious insulin reaction if you do not eat. Conversely, if you are unaware that your blood sugar is precariously high, at, say, 346 mg/dl, you take your insulin injection as usual, and dig into a large meal, followed with a big dessert, then you are not properly controlling your diabetes. In both cases, it is a matter of extreme importance that you know the level of your blood glucose.

There simply are no adequate excuses for not monitoring your blood glucose anymore, but here are a few of the common excuses I have heard many times:

> I am simply not going to test my blood sugar. After all, I do not want another hole stuck in my body.

> No way. That lancet causes too much pain.

> Why should I monitor my blood glucose? What in the world would this data tell me anyway?

> No. I control my diabetes strictly with insulin and exercise.

> I just do not have time for it. It's too much of a hassle.

At one time or another, I have used all of these excuses. I am still very healthy and quite alive and am in excellent shape although I am totally blind. My diabetes is under good control now because I test my blood sugar two or three times every day. You are probably asking yourself, could this guy have saved his eyesight if he had been able to monitor his blood glucose earlier in his diabetic life? Because the nature of diabetes is not fully understood, no endocrinologist or doctor or diabetologist could answer this question with an unequivocal yes or no. But we now have conclusive data from the Diabetes Control and Complications Trial (DCCT), published by the *New England Journal of Medicine* in 1993, that intensive blood glucose control reduces all diabetic complications.

A glucose monitor is an instrument that uses light transmission to read a chemical strip to which a droplet of blood has been applied. When the droplet of blood has reacted adequately with the reagent strip, it is placed into the sample chamber of the device. Depending upon the amount of glucose in the blood, the reagent strip will change color and thus a fairly accurate determination of the blood glucose can be ascertained. The glucose monitor is, then, a miniature spectrophotometer. The reagent strip that has reacted with the sample of blood is placed in front of a light beam within the instrument. The beam measures the amount of glucose in reference to a control established within the electronics of the glucose monitor. When you place the strip in the glucose monitor, you are given a digital reading, therefore arriving at a more accurate actual determination. Reagent strips vary widely in the technique used to apply the blood droplet and the measurement technique used by the instrument.

Some glucose monitors will store results of up to one month's worth of tests, while others require that you keep a logbook for your doctor's review upon your next visit to his or her office. Another clue to how the human mind and especially the diabetic mind works is the following true research story: A test group of diabetic subjects were asked to test their blood sugars for a one-month period, once in the morning and once in the evening, and to write down the results in a special notebook provided to them for this purpose. After the thirty-day period, the results were tabulated. This research project was not intended to see how closely the diabetics kept their blood glucose in control, but to check the honesty of their reporting. The test group had unknowingly been using glucose monitors that retained their blood glucose readings in a special memory. When the actual glucose monitor readings that were stored in memory were compared with the results that were recorded in each diabetic's notebook, the researchers found that almost all of the diabetics had fibbed on reporting their actual test results. I can understand this from my own experience. When reporting my urine sugars as a young diabetic, I hated more than anything to report a high urine sugar rather than a convenient negative sugar amount. Remember, it is only to your advantage to be honest about your true blood glucose level.

Purchase a lancet-holding device and read the instructions that accompany the device. Buy a high-quality blood glucose monitor from one of the reputable companies who manufacture these products for diabetics (see Resource Guide, page 182). I begin by washing my hands thoroughly in warm water with a mild soap. This action helps to stimulate blood flow to the hands and fingers. I have found it best not to use an alcohol pad to clean my fingertip, as this causes the skin to become dry. If you have good blood flow, then you will want to be careful as to the depth of puncture you make by developing your technique and by trying different lancet devices. I let my hand fall to below my waist—this allows the blood flow to be directed to the hands. Then I grasp my finger just below the tip and squeeze it for a few seconds. Then I lance my fingertip to obtain a blood droplet. Really, it is that easy, and soon it becomes second nature, like shaving or trimming one's fingernails.

My first glucose monitor was made by LifeScan. It was the size of a pocket calculator, easy to use, and the first-generation glucose monitor to be produced by this company. They now produce a fine line of glucose monitors and reagent strips. If you want to investigate the LifeScan products for yourself, you will find the LifeScan people very helpful. They produce high-quality products that are durable and long-lasting (see Resource Guide, page 182).

The Diabetes Control and Complications Trial was a ten-year study started in 1984 and devoted to research on diabetics who were stringently controlling their diabetes, that is, attempting to maintain near-normal blood glucose levels of 70–110 mg/dl. Many endocrinologists and diabetologists agree that strict control of the diabetic condition is best managed by self home blood glucose monitoring, careful insulin management, healthy diet, and normal exercise. I will readily admit that it is easy to fudge on the diabetic diet. Eating out, fast food, and social events can sometimes make the diet a little harder to manage. With exercise it seems that we get gung ho about a particular exercise program for a couple of weeks or a couple of months, but then it falls by the wayside. After work, sometimes we are just plain too exhausted to even think of exercising. But, when it comes to insulin injection and blood glucose test time, there should be no fudging and there must always be time. I am trying to talk both honestly and realistically here. As a diabetic myself, I realize that life is full of complexities, time schedules, deadlines, and a great number of other activities to concentrate on rather than diabetes. I feel that testing your blood sugar every day is not an option. It must be thought of in the same regard and level of importance as taking your insulin injections, oral antidiabetic medication, or other medications that must be taken daily. If you can set your mind to this reality early on in your diabetic career, then you will be able to accept it easily.

When I first became diabetic, the only home method we had to determine the relative amount of sugar in our blood was to measure the sugar in our urine. This procedure involved adding ten drops of water to five drops of urine and adding a reactive tablet that produced a color change within a test tube. This color was matched to a chart to indicate the amount of sugar in the urine. The scale went from negative to plus four. Negative meant, of course, no sugar present in the urine. Plus four was that dreaded reading you got after eating three chocolate chip cookies an hour before the test. The trouble with this now-outdated procedure is that the sugar present in the urine is not necessarily a good representation of the true amount of sugar present in the blood. This is due to the renal threshold. In other words, as sugar is spilled out of the blood and into the urine, the percentage of blood glucose may be rising or falling compared to what the urine sugar is actually indicating. If you have taken a dose of insulin, your actual blood sugar may be falling while your urine sugar is still indicating a high percentage of sugar. Theoretically then, if you took additional insulin based on a urine sugar test, while your blood sugar was falling, the extra insulin could plunge you into a dangerous hypoglycemic episode or, simply stated, an insulin reaction. I never did like testing my urine for sugar. It always seemed like an antiquated procedure. I would be stunned at times to feel an impending insulin reaction coming on while my urine sugar showed a three or four plus (high) urine sugar.

By testing the capillary blood in the fingertips, we are able to arrive at a very good relative indication of our level of blood sugar. It is only a good "relative" indication of our blood sugar because we are sampling capillary blood from the peripheral vasculature, not venous blood. Venous blood is taken from the vein in your arm by the blood chemistry laboratory where your doctor sends you periodically for a routine blood test. This laboratory test is a fasting blood sugar (you fast by not ingesting any food for about eight hours before the test), and this blood test is a very accurate, reliable representation of your circulating blood sugar. The instruments we use for home use, although very sophisticated for such a small package, are not laboratory-grade instruments, which are much more accurate.

Nevertheless, self home blood glucose monitoring, a blood sugar test on capillary blood taken from the fingertip, is the best way, at the present time anyway, for us to tell where we are as far as our blood sugar is concerned. With consistent blood glucose monitoring, we can see trends in daily blood sugars. This will assist your doctor in arriving at proper insulin dose alterations for you. It also allows you to control your diabetes on a day-to-day basis better than ever before.

The lancet that you use to prick your finger is razor sharp and creates a microfine hole from which to obtain a single droplet of blood for application onto the reagent strip. This is indeed a very small hole that is made in the fingertip. However, it can and does smart a little at times. Is it a major deal or huge calamity? No, I do not think so. It is but a minor irritation that, with time, technique, and patience, can easily be gotten used to and really not even noticed anymore, although at first the lancet and the bloodletting may not be so easy to take.

I had been a diabetic for many years before self home blood glucose monitoring came into the picture. When it came time for me to begin testing my blood sugar, it was almost ten times harder for me to use the lancet on myself to obtain a tiny drop of blood from my fingertip than anything I could remember at the time. I carefully analyzed my situation with a fellow diabetic who was a pharmacist. He had lost his older brother to diabetes, with complications of blindness and kidney disease, so he tried to maintain strict control of his diabetes. His uncle, also a diabetic, was complaining that the prick of the fingertip in order to obtain a blood sample was just too painful. The pharmacist said to his uncle, "What a bunch of crap! How can a little finger prick that is felt for only a few seconds bother a tough Green Beret like yourself?" If you feel a little intimidated over the lancet and drop of blood, do not let it bother you one bit. Just know that many others have felt and do feel exactly the same way. And remember also, do not sweat the small stuff. The tremendous benefits you will derive from better control of your diabetes far outweighs the minor inconvenience of checking your blood sugar regularly.

5

Clinical Blood Tests

As diabetics, we know the importance of self home blood glucose monitoring on a daily basis to inform us of how well we are utilizing insulin or oral antidiabetic medication, diet, and exercise, but a finger capillary blood sample is not as accurate a determination of actual blood glucose as is circulating venous blood taken from a vein in the arm. This blood sample is what a diagnostic laboratory examines when your doctor orders a routine blood chemistry, including a fasting blood glucose. I suggest you have a routine blood chemistry performed, with fasting blood glucose, triglycerides, both high- and low-density lipoproteins for your total cholesterol measurement, and a glycated hemoglobin, every four months, or at the very least, every six months. This will accomplish two very important things. First it will provide you and your doctor with vital information on the real status of your diabetic condition and your health in general, and second it will force you to visit your doctor on a regular basis. Always keep in mind that the best diabetes management program includes good communication with your doctor. Your health care team is there to provide the best approach to managing your diabetes. It is your responsibility to evaluate good sound advice, practice good diabetes techniques, and become better educated in the knowledge that is available on this tremendously complex subject.

When I have a routine blood chemistry performed, I ask for a complete blood chemistry, a glycated hemoglobin (called a hemoglobin A_1C, Hb A_1C), a fasting blood chemistry, a total cholesterol including high-density lipoprotein (HDL) and low-density lipoprotein (LDL) fractions, and others as my doctor advises.

The following is a breakdown of the clinical laboratory blood chemistry tests that your doctor may order for you.

White blood cell count
Abbreviation: WBC
Normal value: 500–11,000/cu mm

May indicate problems with: kidney, pancreas, heart, liver, lung. This test tells how many infection-fighting cells, white blood cells, are present in the blood. Low levels of white blood cells indicate too few infection-fighting cells, while high levels indicate you may have an infection. Some medications, such as Imuran, may change results of the white blood cell count. Drugs like prednisone may elevate the WBC count.

Hematocrit
Abbreviation: HCT
Normal Value: 36.0–46.0 percent

May indicate problems with: kidney, heart, pancreas, liver, lung. This test tells how many oxygen-carrying red blood cells are in the blood. A low level can make you anemic, tired, and short of breath, while high levels can make your blood thicker and cause problems with clotting. A lot of bleeding can make the hemotocrit go down, while blood transfusions make the hematocrit go up.

Platelets
Abbreviation: PLT
Normal value: 150,000–350,000/cu mm

May indicate problems with: kidney, pancreas, liver, heart, lung. This test tells how many cells that make the blood clot are in the blood. A low-level platelet result indicates you may bleed more easily, while high levels may make your blood very thick and require use of a blood-thinning agent. Liver disease and some medications can change results of the platelet count.

Potassium
Abbreviation: K+
Normal value: 3.5–5.0 mEq/l

May indicate problems with: kidney, pancreas, liver, heart, lung. This test tells how much potassium is in the blood. Potassium helps the heart and makes other muscles work well. High levels of potassium may indicate possible problems with the heartbeat and too much acid in the blood. Low levels may indicate possible problems with the heartbeat. Kidney failure can increase the level of potassium in the blood, as can high levels of acid. Because high acidity and high potassium levels are seen in the case of pancreas transplants, sodium bicarbonate is used to lower this level. The use of diuretics can also cause low levels of potassium.

Carbon Dioxide
Abbreviation: CO_2
Normal value: 24–30 mEq/l

May indicate problems with: kidney, pancreas, heart, liver, lung. This test reflects the acid balance in your blood. Low levels of CO_2 mean too much acid is in the blood. This makes you feel tired and short of breath. Kidney failure or pancreas transplants can cause CO_2 levels to fall. The CO_2 level is increased by taking sodium bicarbonate tablets.

The following two tests are used to assess kidney functioning.

Blood Urea Nitrogen
Abbreviation: BUN
Normal value: 7–22 mg/dl

Creatinine
Abbreviation: CR
Normal value: 0.5–1.2 mg/dl

Both of these tests may indicate problems with kidney, pancreas, liver, heart, and lung. High BUN levels may mean that the kidney is not functioning well. High levels may mean that the kidney is actually in kidney failure; high drug levels of cyclosporine (an anti-rejection drug) and tacrolimus (another antirejection drug) may indicate organ rejection. The BUN level may also be increased by a diet high in protein.

Magnesium
Abbreviation: Mg
Normal value: 1.3–2.0 mEq/l

May indicate problems with: kidney, pancreas, liver, heart, lung. This test tells how much magnesium is present in the blood. Your body needs magnesium in order to carry out many vital functions including heart rate. Low levels of magnesium can cause muscle weakness, sleepiness, and problems with the heartbeat. Medicines like cyclosporine and tacrolimus can cause your magnesium level to go down. By taking magnesium oxide tablets, you can keep your magnesium level normal. The antibiotic trade named Cipro can cause poor absorption of magnesium, so it should be taken two hours prior to taking magnesium.

Total and Direct Bilirubin
Normal value: 0.2–1.2 mg/dl total, 0.0–0.4 mg/dl direct

May indicate problems with: pancreas, liver, heart, lung.

This test tells how well the liver is working. High levels may mean that the liver is not working well. Liver failure causes the levels to rise as a sick liver cannot remove the bilirubin, which is a waste product, from the blood.

The following liver enzyme tests are generally conducted as a group.

AST or SGOT
Normal value: 0–35 IU/l

ALT or SGPT
Normal value: 0–31 IU/l

ALK PHOSP
Normal value: 30–120 IU/l

GGT
Normal value: 8–51 IU/l

LDH
Normal value: 0–220 IU/l

These five tests tell whether there may be damage to the liver, heart, or bone. They may also indicate problems with kidney, heart, pancreas, liver, and lung. A high level means that the enzyme being tested is released into the blood, as it would be if there were damage to the liver, heart, or bone. This damage can be a result of a transplant organ rejection or as a response to certain medicines. Liver failure increases these enzyme levels, especially ALT and GGT. The bone disease that occurs with kidney failure can increase the ALK PHOSP. Certain medicines such as imuran can cause AST and ALT to rise.

The following two tests are generally conducted together.

PT
Normal value: 11.2–13.6 sec

PTT
Normal value: 20–31.6 sec

These tests are used to determine the clotting function of the blood. They may indicate problems with liver, heart, and lung. A high level of PTT may mean that your blood is unable to clot. Liver failure and some medicines can cause this problem. Liver failure can cause your blood to not clot well, and medicines like coumadin and heparin, used to thin the blood, may cause high levels.

Which of the following two tests is administered depends on the antirejection drug that is being taken by the patient.

Cyclosporine Level
Normal value in whole blood HPLC: 150–300 ng/ml

Tacrolimus Level
Normal whole blood TDX level: 6–15 ng/ml

These tests tell how much cyclosporine or tacrolimus is in the blood. Both of these medicines are used to prevent tissue rejection. These tests may indicate problems with kidney, pancreas, liver, heart, and lung. Low levels of these drugs can increase the risk of rejection, while high levels can cause other problems in organs such as the kidneys and can increase the chance of infection. Always have your blood drawn twelve hours after the last dose for the best test results, based on a twice-a-day dosing regiment. Having the blood drawn earlier may make the result high; later may make it low.

Glucose
Blood Sugar
Normal fasting level: 70–115 mg/dl

May indicate problems with: liver, kidney, pancreas, heart, lungs.

A fasting blood sugar tells how well you control your diabetes. It can also tell how well a transplanted pancreas is working. High blood glucose levels can cause problems such as excessive thirst, fatigue, hunger, and weight loss. It can also mean that your transplanted pancreas is not working as well as it should. Low blood glucose levels can make you feel faint, causing sweating, nervousness, fast pulse, and headache. Acute stress such as surgery or infection, intravenous fluids with sugar, steroids, and pancreas transplants can all cause blood glucose levels to rise. Too much insulin can cause the glucose level to be too low; exercise, severe cold, high fever, and a poor diet can all lower the blood sugar level.

Cholesterol
A fatlike substance
Normal value: Less than 200 mg/dl

May indicate problems with: kidney, pancreas, liver, heart, lungs.

This test indicates whether there is a problem with liver function and if you are at a higher risk for having a heart attack. A high cholesterol level can cause narrowing or blockage of blood vessels, which may lead to a heart attack or stroke. When the liver does not function well, the cholesterol level may be low. A high level may be caused by eating fatty foods twelve hours before taking your blood test; therefore, it is best to fast for ten hours before your blood is drawn. Diabetes and some other diseases cause elevated cholesterol levels. Certain medicines, such as prednisone and cyclosporine, may increase the level. A healthy, low-fat diet and exercise will lower cholesterol levels. Bile-duct blockage can cause a high level.

Urine Culture

Indicates the presence of bacteria, caused by an infection, in your urine. This test may indicate problems with kidney and pancreas. An infection in the urine can cause a burning sensation when you urinate, more frequent urination, and a change in color and odor of your urine. In order to obtain an accurate result for a urine culture test, it is important to clean yourself well before providing the sample.

Urine Amylase

This test can tell how well a transplanted pancreas is working. A high level of urine amylase may mean that the transplanted pancreas is making enough amylase and working well. A low level may mean the first sign of rejection of the transplanted pancreas. High levels may be caused by certain medications or inflammation of the pancreas. An obstruction of the pancreatic duct may result in a low level of amylase.

Glycated Hemoglobin

A very important clinical blood test for the diabetic is a glycated, or glycosylated, hemoglobin (GHb) or hemoglobin A_1C (Hb A_1C). It has become the most important tool in ascertaining your level of blood glucose control. Hemoglobin is the red respiratory protein of erythrocytes, the red blood cells. It transports oxygen, in the form of oxyhemoglobin, HbO_2, from the lungs to the tissues where the oxygen is readily released. Glycated hemoglobin is a generic term for hemoglobin that contains glucose or some other carbohydrate.

This test tells how well you have controlled your blood glucose for the last 120 days and is based on the life of the red blood cell

(RBC). The RBC is freely permeable to glucose, and the amount of glucose that enters the RBC is dependent on the concentration of glucose that enters the RBC over its 120-day life span. Glucose within the RBC combines with hemoglobin A in a two-step process. The chemistry involved here is quite elegant and complicated. However, modern clinical chemistry takes advantage of the natural processes in order to provide us diabetics with better diagnostic information as to how well we are actually controlling our blood sugar level. The Hb A_1C test is measured as a percentage. For instance, if your measured value is determined to be 6 percent, this means that for the preceding 120 days, your blood glucose averaged approximately 114 mg/dl on a daily basis. Because this is in the normal range, this value is considered excellent control of your diabetes. If your Hb A_1C value were determined to be 10 percent, then this value would be equivalent to 247 mg/dl, thus not as good control on a daily basis. The Health and Public Policy Committee of the American College of Physicians recommends that the Hb A_1C test be performed four times per year for the Type I insulin-dependent diabetic and two times per year in those with Type II non-insulin-dependent diabetes. Exceptions to this general guideline are for those who are utilizing intensive insulin therapy, including multiple injections or an internal insulin pump, or those who may have undergone a major change in diabetes therapy.

This brief chapter on clinical blood chemistry is designed to help you better understand your test results and better appreciate your doctor's expertise as he or she recommends a course of action designed to help you keep your diabetes under the best control.

6

New Treatment Modalities

The theory and practice of diabetes management have vastly changed over the years. A major breakthrough was the discovery of insulin in 1922. Some of the improvements, small but important modifications, include the disposable syringe rather than the glass syringes I remember when I was young, and the miniature spectrophotometer, which has replaced the clumsy method of urine sugar testing and has made self home blood glucose monitoring one of the most significant contributions in the control of diabetes. This clever little instrument can fit in the palm of the hand or can be carried like a fountain pen in a pocket. There have been great strides in the purification techniques used in the modern-day production of insulin, and the new oral antidiabetic medications hold great promise for the future. During your lifetime as a diabetic, you will probably see incredible discoveries made in the advancement of the understanding of diabetes. In the long history of this disease, better and better ways to manage it are being developed all the time, but an ultimate cure seems as far away as ever. Nondiabetics often do not realize that insulin is only a management tool, not a cure. Your own knowledge base is one of your most important assets in the successful management of diabetes.

In understanding diabetes, the theory of its organic origins has changed over the years. When I was first diagnosed thirty-two years ago, doctors looked closely for a genetic link as the reason for my developing this disease. Over the years, doctors have searched for viral clues as to the origin of diabetes in patients who have no genetic link to the disease. This has proved to be a difficult search. However, it is felt today that if a young person who is diagnosed to be prediabetic can be treated with antirejection drug therapy, then perhaps the pancreas can be saved from destroying itself by mechanisms not presently understood. It is in this vein that current research is proceeding to unravel the autoimmune theory of diabetes and other metabolic diseases. It is thought by some researchers that when first developing diabetes, it is this autoimmune response that destroys the insulin-producing cells within the pancreas. In a recent collaborative study reported at the International Diabetes Federation Congress by Dr. Jean Francois Bach, professor of Immunology at the Sorbonne Institute in Paris, it was determined that early immunosuppression drug therapy restores beta-cell function and delays onset of Type I insulin-dependent diabetes. In this five-year study, involving over six hundred patients, a team of investigators found that cyclosporine delays the autoimmune process. The impact of this finding, which is said to be "without a doubt," is vitally important to those young people who are destined to become tomorrow's diabetics. From 30 to 50 percent of immunosuppressant-treated patients incurred remission from beta-cell destruction (from diabetes) that lasted from two to four years. The patients in this group also showed the same excellent metabolic control as the patients on insulin only, and they required less insulin upon relapse. Findings indicate that the earlier immunosuppression therapy is begun, the higher the remission rate and the better the metabolic control. After some years with diabetes, some key organs, such as the eyes and kidneys, are especially prone to whatever factors are turned on in the autoimmune response. As research proceeds at a frantic pace to understand AIDS (acquired immune deficiency syndrome), spin-off benefits, such as the better understanding of cancer and diabetes, will certainly ensue. A major worldwide effort is being expended at this time in order to better understand the mystery of the autoimmune response in human beings.

When looking for a doctor to manage your diabetes, you will find that most general practitioners and family practice doctors will have a feel for the management techniques used in good clinical practice today, although some may not know a great deal about diabetes specifically. You want a doctor who is not only a good diagnostician and clinician, but also a good teacher and, most important, a good learner and listener. Therefore, if your doctor does not presently have a lot of experience with diabetic patients, then it will be up to him or her to become current in modern-day therapy techniques in order to best help you manage your diabetes. And it will be your task to do the best possible job in following your doctor's orders and to try to comply with his or her recommendations for your best health.

One of the tough old internal medicine professors in medical school always asked his students, "What is the biggest problem in diabetes?" Many students fail to answer this question correctly. The answer, well known to anyone in medical practice, is "Patient compliance." Problems with compliance by the diabetic patient go back a long way. Most doctors will tell you that getting a patient to comply with his or her best advice is a tremendously difficult job. A doctor can advise until he or she is blue in the face that a diabetic's smoking is fatalistic and stupid, but if the diabetic wishes not to comply, then there is nothing for the doctor to do but watch the progressive nature of diabetes take its even more progressive and insidious route to destruction, with the deleterious nature of smoking added in.

Smoking can pose a potential risk. Details from a study on a population of over forty thousand men indicate that one-pack-a-day smokers are twice as likely as nonsmokers to develop Type II non-insulin-dependent diabetes. Moderate drinkers have a lowered tendency to develop Type II diabetes than do those who abstain. Clearly, the message to smokers is to stop. Additionally, they should have a routine fasting blood chemistry test because studies carried out by Stanford endocrinologist Jerrold Reven showed that chronic smokers develop a defect in their sugar metabolism, a clue to the potential of future, impending diabetes.

When you provide your doctor with an abundance of information about yourself, you are helping your doctor make better-informed decisions about the management steps he or she should advise you to proceed with and carry out. For instance, if you kept a running log of every day's blood glucose values, the time you checked your blood sugar, reaction times, notes of overeating or the piece of cherry pie you snitched, and so on, then your doctor would be able to better evaluate your daily routine with your diabetes. Contrast this example with the diabetic who, when asked how his blood sugars are running, answers, "Well, they are just fine." If the doctor has to forcefully pry this information from you, both of you most probably will become frustrated. If your doctor recommends that you monitor your blood glucose three times a day in order to establish a baseline, and you do not take this advice, who are you really hurting?

When I was first diagnosed, I was instructed to give myself one insulin injection per day composed of a mixture of short-acting regular insulin and intermediate-acting insulin in an amount that would control my blood sugar over a twenty-four-hour period. Not too many years after that, doctors treating insulin-dependent diabetics began advising the two-shot-per-day program. In this method, an additional injection of insulin was to be given before the evening meal, usually in a much smaller amount than the morning injection. Many insulin-dependent diabetics today are using the two-injection method, which has proved to be very successful, due in part to the advent of home self blood glucose monitoring.

About ten years ago, the four-injection method of tight control became popular among endocrinologists and diabetologists. In this method, an injection of regular insulin is given approximately every six hours. This means that you must check your blood sugar once every six hours, or four times per day, at the minimum. Because the regular insulin is fast-acting and peaks over a relatively short period of time, one's blood glucose must be carefully monitored to safeguard against hypo- and hyperglycemia. This form of management must be carefully worked out with your doctor and requires a commitment to your diabetes.

Much the same holds when wearing an insulin infusion pump. This method more closely approximates the normal condition, wherein insulin is provided at times where one would expect a high glucose volume, that is, after meals. Use of the insulin pump is the focus of maintaining good glycemic control at the Joslin Diabetes Clinic in Boston, Massachusetts, which operates on the belief that tight blood glucose control and strict management of insulin therapy, diet, and exercise are the only possible choices in dealing with a lifetime of diabetes, a conclusion confirmed by the publication of the results of the ten-year Diabetes Control and Complications Trial in 1993. I believe in tight blood sugar control, with you controlling the diabetes and not the diabetes controlling you.

If I were a newly diagnosed diabetic today, I would give close attention to either the multiple-injection method or the insulin infusion pump. But because I have used the two-injection method for many years, and am now able to closely and tightly control my blood glucose, the four-shot method is not appropriate, as it would be quite difficult to incorporate it into my life as a blind diabetic. You, as a newly diagnosed diabetic, well informed about the problems of not tightly controlling your disease, have more choices than I did when I began. You will have to do some hard thinking about your lifestyle and your personal commitment to diabetes before you will be able to make an intelligent choice.

Home Blood Glucose Monitors

If you have not already read Chapter 4 (page 19) about these important devices that I hope will become an integral part of your everyday fight against diabetes, please do so.

Would you be more inclined to test your blood glucose two, ten, or more times per day if you were not required to lance your finger in order to obtain a blood droplet? I know I certainly would. By using a microsharp lancet, a puncture wound is created by an invasive technique that the diabetic must endure two, four, or more times every day. Think for a moment how nice it would be if there were no lancets involved, no blood to apply to a reagent strip, and, for that matter, no reagent strip either. A new technology is currently being perfected by several companies that will substitute a device using near-infrared (NIR) light energy instead of a lancet. The Futrex Company is now developing a machine that will measure your blood sugar by merely placing your index finger into a hole on the instrument. This small instrument uses NIR light to pass through the skin on the finger to read the glucose level. Near-infrared spectroscopy, when perfected for measuring glucose, will determine the chemical makeup of a person's blood by analyzing the signal changes in the wavelengths of light after it has passed through the tissue. By measuring the glucose-emitted signals, the concentration of sugar levels can be determined. Glucose accounts for only one one-thousandth of the mass of blood, thus making it hard to measure the wavelengths absorbed by glucose, which are also absorbed by other more sizable molecules, including water and fat. The main difficulty in this process is focusing in on those specific wavelengths that, although weakly absorbed by glucose, are even less absorbed by surrounding tissues.

Robert Rosenthal, owner of Futrex, is a Type II diabetic himself and understands the great difference perfecting his noninvasive NIR glucose monitor will make to his own life and to all diabetics. Clinical trials on a diabetic population of over one thousand have been undertaken with diabetic volunteers. These trials measure a diabetic's blood glucose with the new NIR light device; then a comparison measurement is made using a standard blood glucose monitor, which uses a droplet of blood and a reagent strip. The company hopes to be able to calibrate their new device for accuracy, and win Food and Drug Administration approval.

Another interesting noninvasive technology is currently under research at the University of California, San Francisco, and Signus Thereapeutic Corporation, Redwood City, California, to measure glucose levels transdermally, through the skin, with the Gluco-Watch. This process, called reverse iontophoresis, uses a steady electric current to extract glucose molecules from the body, a process originally designed to deliver drugs transdermally by enlarging the pores in order to allow large drug molecules to enter in. Included with this noninvasive monitor is a gluco pad that adheres to the skin. This pad is placed on the back of the Gluco-Watch, which can measure and display the blood glucose value. The pad must be replaced daily; the watch allows for continuous monitoring of glucose levels. This transdermal concept has been considered by such pharmaceutical giants as Eli Lilly, Becton-Dickinson, and the Alza Corporation. With the potential market of over $1.5 billion per year, the race is on to provide the diabetic community with a reliable and affordable noninvasive blood glucose monitoring device that will make all our lives a little easier.

When I first lost my eyesight, there were no manufacturers of blood glucose monitors with speech output. Ames had tried to market a talking glucose monitor in the early 1980s; however, technical problems prevented it from further development. So initially, I could not test my blood sugar by myself and had to rely on help from my family. Voice synthesis technology now enables me to obtain my blood glucose values myself. The digital information from the blood glucose monitor is fed through a data cable into a voice box, where the signal is read out in electronic speech. I have used the meters made by LifeScan, a division of Johnson and Johnson, almost exclusively since the early 1980s. I presently use the LifeScan One Touch Profile blood glucose monitor, the company's newest design and concept for better diabetes management. This meter has easy testing procedures and, along with the One Touch Profile Diabetes Tracking System, enables the diabetic to monitor trends of high and low blood sugars quickly. It also features fourteen- and thirty-day blood glucose averaging, and 250-test memory. You can also keep an accurate history of your insulin dosage. The In Touch Profile Diabetes Management computer software allows connection to a personal computer for reviewing, graphing, and printing blood glucose test results. This beautifully designed instrument is adaptable for use with a voice box. I have found this meter to be the most sophisticated and most accurate meter on the market today.

I try to take my insulin about thirty minutes before a meal, but please remember that this thirty-minute period is only a guideline. You must learn to be flexible with your diabetes and yet still remain within the guidelines as much as possible. Let me illustrate with an example from real life. A diabetic friend considered the guideline of taking insulin thirty minutes before a meal to be a rule that was not to be broken under any circumstances. He would take his insulin injection without checking his blood sugar, and then wait thirty minutes before eating. When I protested that he *must* check his blood sugar, he just shrugged his shoulders and blew it off. I tried logic and my experience with diabetes, and then I resorted to stepping out of my role as friend and into the role of rigid endocrinologist. Nothing would convince him that a blood sugar test before taking his insulin could tell him if his glucose levels were dangerously low, in which case taking his insulin and waiting thirty minutes before eating could prove disastrous. He took an injection, and feeling an insulin reaction coming on, he lay down to rest and never awoke. He was found dead two days later. This was a needless loss of a young person's life. I can only hope that you learn from my experiences and the experiences of others.

Insulin Delivery Systems

The standard syringe is the most important and widely used of the insulin delivery systems. It is convenient, accessible, easy to operate, portable, and fast. It is important to think of your insulin syringes as part of your right arm, or left arm if you are left-handed. The fact is that you cannot leave home without these instruments, which deliver your life-sustaining fluid. I have used an insulin syringe to take my injections on jet liners while on business trips, in a Ferrari with the top down on a pleasure trip, in a rather unclean bathroom in Mexico; these all-important syringes are always with me from classroom to emergency room, from research lab to restaurant, in my coat pocket, shirt pocket, pants pocket, my medical bag, my carry-on luggage.

The disposable insulin syringe can be used several times (for a week's worth of injections), even though it was designed to be used only one time and then thrown away. In a 1983 study that appeared in *Diabetes Care*, a clinicians' journal published by the American Diabetes Association, it was found that the typical insulin syringe was safe to reuse for up to thirty days. You must use good sterile technique in drawing up your insulin and always use an alcohol pad to thoroughly clean your injection site. If as a new diabetic, you train yourself well in using good sterile technique and good insulin syringe and vial handling, and if you are confident about your proficiency, you can certainly benefit monetarily from this idea. A limiting factor to the life of the syringe is the sharpness of the needle. Once the needle is dull, use a fresh syringe. I prefer to reuse a syringe for a week (two injections per day) and then start with a fresh syringe.

This is a useful time to look at the subject of the cost of diabetic treatment. Today the average box of one hundred insulin syringes is about twenty-five dollars. I use approximately one thousand syringes per year and therefore buy them by the thousand because I get a better price. I use disposable alcohol pads for each injection; these are available for three or four dollars per hundred. The two different insulin preparations I use cost about fifteen dollars per vial, and I use about one vial of each type per month.

My first glucose monitor cost about five hundred dollars. Due to their wide acceptability and importance, the cost of these units has dropped drastically. I suggest you buy a high-quality glucose monitor; ask your pharmacist to help you choose one. Test strips for the glucose monitor run approximately sixty dollars per hundred, so they are a constant high-cost item. Because I do two to three tests per day, the one-hundred-count bottle of strips lasts me approximately one month.

The initial cost of a lancet device for finger piercing runs about twenty-five dollars and should be of high quality, as it will be used every day. The lancets are about five dollars per hundred. I use a fresh lancet each time, using two or three per day.

When you add all this up, it is no wonder that the diabetic supplies market is a multibillion-dollar industry for the home blood glucose monitoring segment alone. Diabetes is an expensive disease, but it is in your interest to do the best you can in obtaining the best-quality products to manage your disease. I have figured my current diabetic supplies cost to be approximately $250 per month. With a group medical plan, your costs might be much less.

Another insulin delivery system is the jet injection system. In this system there is no needle; the insulin penetrates the skin by way of a high-pressure air blast. The military tested air jet injection systems back in the early sixties to do mass inoculations for military troops and dependents. I know because I was a military dependent at that time and remember only too well waiting in line to get a shot by air injection. Most of the kids did not know whether to cry because the air blast was uncomfortable or to be happy because there were no hideous-looking needles to be stabbed into their arms. You need to remember that the air jet injection is an invasive technique. There is a penetration of the skin and there will be some slight feeling involved. As you become more proficient in your technique, you will feel less pain with jet injection than with a standard syringe injection.

For some diabetics the jet injection system is not advisable. If you have a bleeding disorder, such as hemophilia, that involves a low platelet count, or if you are too thin, or have little or no strength in your hands, or have arthritis of the hands or wrists, or have low vision or blindness, you are advised not to use jet injectors. Also, use of any of the jet injection systems available requires patience, training, and willingness to comply with the requirements of using a high-tech instrument.

The Medi Jector Jet Injector system by Medi-Ject Corporation has pioneered the technology of air injection for the diabetic insulin-dependent population for many years. Presently, there are two basic models of air injection syringe from Medi-Ject. The larger unit is capable of delivering more than fifty units of insulin, whereas the lower-dose model is restricted to fifty units and below. Use of the jet injector requires commitment, attention to detail, and a willingness to learn and develop a new technique.

Because low vision or blindness prevents normal use of the jet injector, I decided to try this system after I became totally blind in 1985 in order to prove to myself that I could use an instrument that was designed primarily for the sighted diabetic. I attended a training course set up by Medi-Ject Corporation. I persevered in the use of the jet injector and spent time discussing the benefits on the phone with a member of their excellent support staff. There are, today, a number of totally blind diabetic users of the Medi Jector Jet Injector system, which says a lot for the diabetic who chooses to use this high-tech delivery system as well as for the Medi-Ject personnel who provide guidance and help with any problems.

The Medi Jector must be meticulously cleaned every two weeks because insulin is a rather viscous, sticky fluid. This means disassembling the barrel, plunger, and nozzle and sterilizing all the parts in boiling water for at least twenty minutes. If for some reason the Medi Jector is not used every day, the cleaning procedure must be done more often. When using the Medi Jector, you must check your blood sugar at least once per day.

What are the benefits of using jet injection systems? There have been many studies supporting the fact that after many years of standard insulin injections, the absorption of the injected insulin slows down in the areas of injected tissue and thus uniform dispersement of the insulin does not take place. This so-called insulin pooling effect can cause a delay in the onset of insulin due to slowed insulin absorption. The jet injector blasts the insulin into the injection site in a uniform dispersant pattern, therefore aiding in the absorption of the insulin dose. This is said to be easier on the tissue at the injection site and thus improves the control of one's diabetes. It has also been reported that use of the Medi Jector tends to reduce insulin antibody formation because the Medi Jector injects insulin via a fine jet dispersal system, thereby increasing the insulin absorption rate. Insulin antibodies tend to cause a resistance to the uptake of insulin at the cellular level, thus creating the need for additional insulin, which in turn creates more insulin resistance. Results of a study carried out at the Samsung Research Clinic in Santa Barbara in the 1980s on pregnant women who had developed gestational diabetes seem to show that the Medi Jector lowered insulin antibody formation.

Another possible benefit of use of jet injection systems is patient compliance. Because some diabetics will not follow their doctors' orders to take two or more insulin injections per day, use of the Medi Jector has shown improvement in those diabetics who desire to better control their disease.

An additional benefit to using the jet injector is the ability to inject sites that are inaccessible with an ordinary syringe. Once the jet injector is loaded with your insulin dose, it is placed firmly against the skin at the chosen injection site. Then, to discharge the injector, all you do is press the discharge button located at the top of the instrument. Especially in the case of the young diabetic child, the jet injector can be useful in preventing lipodystrophy, disruption of the fat layer found beneath the skin. This condition is a serious consideration for all diabetics who use insulin. By not using a needle, the Medi Jector is believed to help in the prevention of the tendency to damage fat and skin tissue. An added benefit is the dispersal action of the air injection itself.

Another insulin delivery system is the insulin pump. The modern insulin pump is a marvel of high-tech ingenuity and design. The new pumps are approximately the overall dimensions of a credit card, but thicker. The electronics contain microminiature computer circuits so that you can program the pump to deliver insulin doses during peak blood sugar times, and then very small doses during the day, so that blood sugar is kept to near-normal levels throughout the entire twenty-four-hour period. The base rate, or basal rate, is the programmed rate of insulin delivery based on your specific metabolic requirements. The extra dose given before a meal or a little extra dessert, based on your blood glucose reading, is called the *bolus dose.* How do you know if your pump is delivering enough insulin or too much insulin? You will need to test your blood sugar at least four to six times per day when using an insulin pump.

I want to make perfectly clear that insulin-pump therapy does not provide better control than standard insulin therapy. A pump in use today can do only what the user tells the pump to do by way of programming it. The insulin pump delivery system demands an above-average desire to control your diabetes to the utmost in our present technology base. In order to accomplish this, you must be willing to do an above-average job in managing your diabetes. This represents a therapeutic interaction on your part as the intelligent diabetic so that the insulin pump can maximize your insulin delivery for the most efficient utilization. I want to stress the point that the insulin pump, while providing maximum diabetic control, requires a very real commitment to your diabetes; if you are willing to pay the price of extra commitment in terms of time and energy, then the pump is something you will want to investigate for yourself in consultation with your doctor. The insulin pump requires a few days to calibrate to your particular insulin requirements, diet, and exercise. Additionally, you may have to check your blood sugar many more times per day during this initial start-up time than you will thereafter. However, use of the pump still requires at least four blood sugar tests per day.

The insulin pump uses only regular insulin. Due to the short-acting nature of regular insulin, it provides a better control system when administered in multiple doses throughout a twenty-four-hour period. Very specialized microminiature motors depress the plunger that delivers insulin into a small catheter tube whose needle is placed in the abdomen and secured down with a butterfly bandage. This in-dwelling catheter needle must be changed to a new insertion site location on the abdomen about every three days. Again, good sterile technique is required when administering your catheter procedure. You must carefully avoid an infection at the catheter's needle site. Imagine yourself tethered to a beautiful small instrument by a very small line carrying your life-sustaining insulin. You will sleep with this instrument, eat with it, work with it, in fact, do everything you normally do in life while attached to your insulin pump. The catheter may be removed from the pump itself while taking a shower, swimming, or any other activity where the physical unit must be protected; however, most of the time you will remain attached to the pump. The pump itself can be attached to your belt or any other convenient location where you can have access to programming its functions and monitoring its process.

The newer pumps have audible alarms to signal dangerous conditions such as an occluded catheter or low insulin.

The benefits of using the insulin pump are numerous. I think the most important is that you are closely mimicking the normal insulin delivery system of the normal pancreas through many small doses of insulin maintained throughout the day. By testing your blood sugar, you are acting as an artificial sensor to detect your blood sugar level in order to insure that the continuous infusion of insulin is adequate, not too high or too low. Another advantage to the pump is that you are connected to this instrument on a twenty-four-hour-a-day basis and there is, basically, no time allowed for the convenient denial of the fact that you are a diabetic, something that happens only too frequently with most diabetics. Because of the risk of low-blood-sugar episodes while using the pump, more frequent monitoring of your blood sugar is necessary, which is, in my opinion, a definite benefit. You are acutely aware of your blood sugar at different intervals of the day, and thus in better control.

The most important risk in using the insulin pump is that faced by all diabetics, and that is low blood sugar reactions. Consider that if your blood sugar is plummeting downward, lower and lower, and if you have not checked your blood sugar during the time you are sleeping, with continual infusion of insulin you will be plunged deeper and deeper into hypoglycemia. This is, indeed, a life-threatening situation. If you sleep alone, or if your mate sleeps deeply and does not notice your sweating, moans, and, in severe cases, convulsions, you could be facing an emergency; immediate action is required with sugar-laced orange juice and/or glucagon injection. In severe cases, the Emergency Medical Service (EMS) must be called for administration of intravenous glucose to prevent a coma. Low-blood-sugar reactions happen to all of us who are controlling our blood sugar to at- or near-normal levels. If for some reason your catheter becomes kinked or blocked, then you will not get enough insulin. Because you use only regular insulin in the pump, there is no intermediate or long-lasting insulin to carry you along. If this persists unnoticed by you, you may go into diabetic ketoacidosis, or extremely high blood sugar, which is also a bad situation, although only in the worst prolonged high blood sugar states will coma occur. Therefore, if given the choice, you would prefer to have high blood sugar rather than extremely low blood sugar. Suffice it to say that both high and low blood sugar states must be controlled. Strive for normal blood sugar at all times. By doing this, you will achieve a near-normal situation more times and thus have better control of your diabetes.

Although some blind diabetics are using the insulin pump, I do not use one, although I had planned to just before I lost my eyesight in 1984. There are two well-known manufacturers of insulin pumps. Disetronic produces a very high-tech insulin pump that is manufactured in Switzerland. The Mini Med Insulin pump is a beautiful and well-made product that has been available for over twelve years. (See page 186 for information on these products.)

In the early seventies, Dr. J. Stuart Soeldner at the Joslin Diabetes Clinic pioneered an implantable insulin pump. An extensive study was carried out on the hardware necessary to accomplish the internal administration of insulin by an electromechanical device implanted beneath the skin. At that time, microelectronics was in its infancy. Today, we live in a world where even the electronic fuel injection in cars is controlled by a computer chip. As in the case of the insulin pump worn externally, computer circuitry is vital to the control of the miniature components involved in the pump. Today, experimental clinical trials are being carried out on the implantable insulin pump. This unit is three inches by three inches by one inch thick. It is implanted below the skin in the area of the abdomen. Once the instrument is in place, you control functions by remote control, much like you control your television set. In order to maintain an insulin source, you must inject a month's worth of regular insulin through a membrane on the pump. You inject this large amount of insulin through your skin and into the reservoir located in the pump inside your body. To me this sounds like an artificial pancreas. If this would ultimately work, then how about a system that would automatically monitor the circulating blood glucose and send a signal to the pump to administer a dose of insulin right after you have finished a meal or after you have just eaten a large chocolate chip cookie? The Japanese have worked very hard on this scenario by using platinum electrodes implanted in the body that would monitor the blood glucose. The problem with these electrodes is that platinum is very expensive and the electrodes become clogged up with tissue buildup after about one week. But if a system were to be able to work in this manner, we would achieve a true artificial pancreas loop system that would eliminate a lot of the problems found in diabetes management today. The implantable insulin pump is not FDA approved as yet. A few brave insulin-dependent diabetics are acting as experimental subjects in order to test this new device. Are there dangers involved? You bet there are. In fact, diabetic subjects are very carefully chosen for this preclinical trial and must be prepared for the worst and the best of their particular experimental test results. Suffice it to say that there are grave risks involved. However, if these tests prove successful, important research data can then be better modulated into future units that may become available to the overall diabetic population. And from this we will all benefit.

Insulin delivery by nasal inhalation has been studied for many years. If insulin could be administered in the same manner you inhale an antihistamine, through the nasal passages, would this not be a great insulin delivery system that would eliminate the dreaded syringes and needles? Syringes and needles could take on a secondary role, which would mean a lot fewer problems in managing the associated ritual of injections. Unfortunately, the nasal inhalation route of insulin delivery has proved unsatisfactory for many reasons, the most important of which is the problem with uniformity of dosages. Modern metered dose containers are available today that are helping to make this delivery system come closer and closer to reality. There are also problems associated with the nasal mucosa itself, such as the possibility of long-term inhalation of insulin causing problems in the upper sinuses.

Pancreatic Tissue Transplantation

The transplantation of suitable donor pancreas tissue (usually from a family member) is a radical method of insulin delivery. Once the transplanted pancreatic tissue begins producing insulin, the diabetic is then rendered undiabetic, or "normal." It is now the practice for a team of surgeons to transplant a kidney along with a section of about one third of a donor pancreas. You must be in need of a kidney transplant in the first place to be a candidate for the double organ replacement, although in some very select cases, diabetics who are not in a state of renal insufficiency are becoming candidates for pancreas transplantation.

Many long-term diabetics who have suffered renal failure and who are candidates for a kidney transplant opt for this double surgery. You would have to do a lot of real soul searching and consultation with your doctor in order to reach an intelligent decision in this matter. Many successful pancreas transplants are performed at the University of Minnesota, where the world experts do their particular brand of miracle working. But you should know that about one third of the diabetics who opt for this surgery do not make it through the difficult course this surgery demands, and they die. Remember also that the diabetic who has need of a kidney transplant is usually the long-term diabetic with eighteen or twenty or even more years of insulin dependence. In the past, only diabetics who had suffered blindness and kidney failure were considered for a pancreas transplant. These diabetics were thought to be in rather end-stage condition, having endured two of diabetes' most ravaging complications, so why not try for a "cure" to the culprit that caused it all in the first place?

The microsurgery that is practiced today by doctors in the operating room is so highly advanced and technical that it goes far beyond a discussion that would fit into this book. I mention transplant surgery only as a point of interest and education so that you will be aware of its existence. Naturally, for the newly diagnosed diabetic, this form of insulin delivery is not viable at the present time. In the future, we may see routine pancreas transplants or transplants of donor beta cells into the subject along the portal vein. A major research effort is being conducted into this method and the experimental model has shown some initial success in dogs.

When I was first starting out in my new diabetic life, there were not many choices. We had the choice of U-40 or U-80 glass insulin syringes to match with whatever concentration of insulin our doctor chose for us. I look back at those times and think about how primitive it was. After you have had diabetes for the next twenty or thirty years, what will the systems look like then? It is indeed my hope and prayer that in the next twenty or thirty years, diabetes will have been cured.

Medic Alert Identification

One important point to consider is diabetic identification. I always carry my diabetic medical identification card, my regular identification cards, and current syringe and insulin prescriptions given to me by my doctor (even though it is not necessary to have a doctor's prescription in order to buy syringes at a pharmacy).

I strongly recommend your becoming a member of the Medic Alert Foundation, a nonprofit organization I have belonged to for nearly thirty years. For a small membership fee, you will be placed in their computer system and given an identification card to carry with you at all times. This card has your name, address, and phone number, as well as the name of your primary physician and his or her phone number. The card also lists emergency symptoms and what a person unfamiliar with your condition should do if you're found in this state. Identification bracelets and neck chains are also available with the words MEDIC ALERT on one side of the bracelet. On the reverse side is the toll-free number of the Medic Alert Foundation and your medical condition inscribed on the middle of the bracelet. See page 180 for their toll-free number and address.

7

Long-term Diabetic Complications: An Overview

"People deny reality. They fight against real feelings caused by real circumstances. They build mental worlds of shoulds, oughts, and might have beens. Real changes only begin with real appraisal and acceptance of what is. Only then is realistic action possible." These are the words of David Reynolds, an American exponent of Japanese Morita Psychotherapy, about personal behavior.

Before we begin the following chapters on the complications of long-term diabetes mellitus, it will be important for you to prepare yourself mentally for just a few moments. Clear your mind so that you will be able to understand in a positive manner that what you are about to read is information and knowledge that will set reference points for your better total understanding of this very complex disease. This information and knowledge will be used to educate and better prepare you in the management of your diabetes on a daily basis. By giving yourself the best possible care every day, by checking your blood sugar, by being conscientious of proper medication intake and dose management, and with proper diet and exercise, after you have accrued enough years with diabetes to be called long-term, it is my hope and prayer that you will not have to suffer any of the long-term complications we will be discussing in the next few chapters.

Think for a few minutes about the history of diabetes. It is fairly well understood that human beings were developing and dying from complications of diabetes before the time of the building of the great pyramids. What secrets might lie within the genetic code that predispose a person for diabetes? Might there be some secret to the development of the human species, the basis of which defies our present understanding of human biochemistry and molecular immunology?

Consider that with the further development of modern high-tech medical procedures, the diabetic has been afforded a longer and longer life span. By living longer, the diabetic is now enduring the complications associated with long-term diabetes that he would not have had to endure before due to his early death. Is it not ironic that by living longer with diabetes, a particular set of medical conditions accompanies the changes encountered naturally as one ages and oftentimes combines to devastatingly handicap the diabetic? Interestingly, this is not the universal case with diabetes. Why does not everyone with diabetes go totally blind? Why do not all with diabetes lose kidney function and suffer bilateral leg amputations? Medicine could possibly have more clues to disease parameters if all diabetics fell neatly into the same mold. But diabetes does not affect all who are living with this disease in the same manner. It is true that diabetes is the number-one cause of new blindness within the United States. But not all long-term diabetics suffer total blindness. In fact, many diabetics incur only the natural aging process associated with lens stiffening and thus require the usual remedy, that is, reading glasses or bifocals. Some diabetics will require treatment for retinopathy but only require essential treatment that does not cause severe diminution of their vision. Many diabetics suffer kidney failure as well as diabetic eye disease, making for a one-two punch that makes surviving extremely difficult. I personally know many courageous diabetics who have suffered both complications at the same time. One can search for answers to the "whys" of all of this, but I have yet to find a satisfactory answer, and let me tell you, during my initial stage with total blindness, I had many solitary moments to contemplate diabetes in its entirety.

In the final analysis, it is up to you to carry forward with the most positive attitude and deal with your disease in an enlightened manner on a daily basis. My personal challenge to you is to study these chapters on long-term complications of diabetes while keeping your mind focused on the positive future medical advances that will make these complications extinct. Perhaps you yourself will become motivated to pursue the study of science and medicine in order to accomplish future advances.

8

Long-term Complications
to the Diabetic Eye

Diabetic retinopathy is a progressive disease of the retina found
in the long-term diabetic. Diabetic retinopathy and associated
sequelae account for the number-one cause of new blindness in the
United States. It is difficult for me to discuss diabetic retinopathy
without becoming emotionally involved. After having had better
than normal vision (20/15) for thirty-five years, I suffered a textbook case of proliferative diabetic retinopathy (after living with
diabetes for twenty years); this was a crushing blow to all areas
of my life. It was, and sometimes still is, difficult for me to accept
total blindness. However, I have been fortunate enough to regain
a high standard of quality of life, and although it may seem hard
to believe, many areas of my life have actually improved over my
sighted life.

Please do not take on an attitude of denial and look at this information as fatalistic or too depressing to read. If you are not psychologically prepared to read about diabetic eye disease at this time,
skip the next few chapters and come back to them when you are
more comfortable in learning about this particular area within the
health of the diabetic.

Before we enter into a discussion of diabetic retinopathy, let's
look briefly at some basic anatomy of the eye itself. Seemingly
unending in complexity in form and function, vision is a miraculous phenomenon of events enabling us to discern detail and
dimension, perspective, color, and motion all at the same time.
Within the intricate bundles of nerves that connect the eye to the
brain lies the future of our better understanding of the true nature
of sight. The eye is so beautiful in its form, so fantastic in its func-

tion, so complex in its intricacy, that it is no wonder that we tend to take it for granted.

The optic nerves are actually tracts of the brain that run alongside the central artery of the retina, a branch of the ophthalmic artery. Vascularly, the ophthalmic artery is a branch of the internal carotid artery and enters the orbit through the optic canal just beneath the optic nerve. The retina is supplied with its blood flow via the internal carotid artery, which branches to the ophthalmic branch and feeds the retina via the central artery of the retina.

Embryologically, the eyeball itself is formed as an outgrowth of the brain, and the two layers of the retina of the adult eye are actually an extension of the brain. If you think about this for just a moment, it makes logical sense that the eye should derive from the exceedingly complex structure of the brain during embryological development. The visual field is focused onto the retina by inversion of the eye. The retina is an electrical transducer of sorts, as it changes electromagnetic radiation into electrical impulses. It is the visual cortex within the brain that is able to decode these electrical impulses to form visual images. The eyeball itself is covered with a tough fibrous coat, which makes it quite durable. It is a fluid-filled cavity that maintains its shape by distributing its hydraulic pressure uniformly.

The outer shell of the eye is composed of the sclera and cornea, making up the fibrous tunic. The white of the eye is called the sclera, from the Greek word *sclerose*, for *hard*. The sclera comprises about 83 percent of the eyeball and provides insertion for the extraocular muscles. Composed of dense connective tissue, the anterior portion of the sclera is covered by the conjunctiva. Containing a great number of small blood vessels and nerve endings, the conjunctiva is the clear covering at the front of the eye. The sclera joins the cornea at the limbus, and the clear cornea comprises about 17 percent of the eyeball. The cornea is composed of dense, regularly arranged collagen fibers, and it is the extreme regularity of the fibers of the tissue that results in the liquid crystalline structure that is completely transparent to light.

The choroid layer is part of the internal vascular tunic of the eye. The choroid layer consists primarily of blood vessels whose blood supply is fed by the short ciliary artery and drained by the vorticose vein. The ciliary layer is the continuation of the forward portion of the choroid layer. It is the ciliary body that suspends the lens with a network of specialized fibers that insert into the capsule of the lens in the front of the eye.

The iris arises from the ciliary body at the front of the eye and divides the space between the cornea and lens into anterior (front) and posterior (back) chambers. Epithelial cells of the ciliary body secrete aqueous humor (liquid) into the posterior chamber.

The optic vesicle (a very small vessel), which, again, is brainlike tissue, forms the retina. There are two primitive layers of the retina, the anterior primitive layer and the posterior primitive layer. The neural retina is the anterior primitive layer. It consists of four major layers of nerves and supporting cells through which light rays must pass to reach the photosensitive cells. These layers are

1. the first layer, consisting of nerve axons that collect at the optic disc, or blind spot of the eye, and pass through a plate in the sclera to form the optic nerve.
2. the second layer, composed of so-called nerve ganglion cells, equivalent to a brain-stem nucleus.
3. the third layer, composed of bipolar cells, equivalent to dorsal root ganglion, another specialized nerve cell.
4. the fourth layer, containing the light-sensitive cells, called rods and cones. Maximum visual acuity is attained at the fovea centralis, where large numbers of cones are concentrated and are at the center of the visual field.

The posterior primitive layer is composed of heavily pigmented retinal cells. It is heavily pigmented in order to absorb any light that passes completely through the anterior layer, the neural retina.

Clinically speaking, retinal detachment is due to separation of the anterior and posterior layers of the retina. Usually, the separation begins at the frontal, anterior, layer, and therefore is usually unnoticed until retinal detachment is well advanced. Interestingly, there is a predisposition for retinal detachment to occur bilaterally, that is, in both eyes, so extreme care must be taken that both eyes do not become seriously compromised. This can certainly be the case in diabetic retinopathy, wherein one eye becomes compromised, and through unique communication pathways, the other eye begins to deteriorate or show signs of damage also. Thankfully, retinal layers may be reattached via photo coagulation procedures (see laser discussion below).

Papilledema is edema, swelling, of the optic disc. This condition may or may not be concomitant with diabetic retinopathy. Papilledema can be observed by ophthalmoscopic examination. The retinal arteries are the only arteries within the body that can be examined directly for signs of hypertension and diabetes using an ophthalmoscope. Many times the suspicion of diabetes is made by an ophthalmologist or optometrist while performing a routine eye exam.

We will briefly discuss the chambers of the eye, and then proceed on to the general discussion of diabetic retinopathy. The anterior chamber of the eye lies between the iris and the cornea. The posterior chamber lies between the iris and the lens, and both chambers contain a thin watery solution called aqueous humor. The vitreous body is a transparent and semigelatinous material and fills the vitreous chamber, which is located just behind the lens. It is, therefore, the lens that separates the aqueous humor from the vitreous body. The vitreous humor is composed of highly ordered and regularly spaced connective tissue cells, thus making it transparent to the transmission of light.

The risk of blindness within the diabetic population increases with age; the risk of blindness seems to be greatest particularly for those diabetics who have retinopathy between the ages of thirty and fifty. Despite these figures, diabetic retinopathy does not lead directly to blindness; many diabetics with retinopathy are able to see quite well. It is proliferative retinopathy and neovascularization, that is, the abundant new growth of blood vessels stemming from the retina, that lead directly to blindness within the majority of the diabetic population who are diagnosed with this condition. The survival time of usable vision after the first lesion appears in diabetic proliferative retinopathy which then proceeds to blindness is only about six years. I find these figures to be distressingly oppressive, since I have witnessed the devastating effects blindness has on the diabetic. As one might guess, other vascular problems are also beginning to appear just when the diabetic is facing losing eyesight.

Although diabetes accounts for the number-one cause of new

blindness in this country, not all diabetics, either Type I or Type II, will lose their eyesight to this complication. Some may incur a slight loss of vision due to retinopathy in its nonproliferative stage, while others may suffer total blindness due to retinopathy in its proliferative stage accompanied by neovascularization. Each case of diabetes is individual and unique, so no one really knows what your long-term case of diabetes will prove to be.

What does this mean for you? Well, consider again the fact that in the days before the discovery of insulin, the complication of diabetic retinopathy was virtually unknown and there were few, if any, cases of diabetic blindness. With the discovery of insulin in 1921, the diabetic population was afforded a longer life span, and thus the increasing tendency for long-term diabetics to live long enough to experience complications of long-term vascular disease and the deterioration of delicate vasculature in organs such as the eye and kidney.

Diabetic retinopathy is broken down into two separate categories. The more benign type of retinopathy is called nonproliferative retinopathy. The more severe retinopathy is called proliferative retinopathy. Many times a diabetic is diagnosed as having the disease when an optometrist or ophthalmologist does a routine eye exam with an ophthalmoscope and finds background nonproliferative retinopathy. Researchers have found that this type of nonproliferative retinopathy is prevalent in insulin-dependent diabetics at the rate of 10 percent after ten years with the disease, 50 percent after the first fifteen years, and 90 percent after twenty-five years' experience with diabetes. So it is clear that retinopathy is a complication associated with many years with diabetes. Proliferative diabetic retinopathy is usually associated with other progressive, insidious diabetic disease complications such as diabetic nephropathy, or diabetic kidney disease, and coronary artery disease.

Proliferative retinopathy causes a host of associated complications that lead almost inevitably to loss of sight, one of the most traumatic complications associated with diabetes. Complications such as neovascularization leads to vitreous hemorrhage and proliferation of fibrous tissue banding. Contraction of this fibrous tissue and weak vasculature proceed to traction retinal detachment, causing additional bleeding into the vitreous. This proliferative retinopathy, medically termed retinitis proliferans, sets up the progressively more and more complicated biochemistry and physical degradation resulting in the very poor prognosis for the retention of useful vision.

Neovascularization arises from the optic disk and surface of the retina. These new vessels are weak and form a circular or loop configuration. As these new vessels add additional weight to the retina, which is already vascularly compromised, the traction on the retina causes a pulling-forward action that can result in partial or total detachment. At this stage, the eye is gravely compromised and the prognosis for the retention of vision is certainly in question. The traction stress on the vitreal retinal vessels eventually causes these vessels to hemorrhage, thus filling the vitreal space with additional blood. Remember, the vitreous humor is the clear jellylike fluid that fills the space between the retina, at the back of the eye, and the lens, located near the front of the eye. When vitreous hemorrhage occurs, this new blood sets up further complications within the eye, one of which is the fact that the vitreous jelly is no longer clear. As the hemorrhage continues unabated, the difficulty of seeing clear images through the vitreous humor becomes greater and greater. This condition also makes it difficult for the treating ophthalmologist to see into the back of the eye.

One of the most successful treatments for diabetic retinopathy is pan-retinal photocoagulation, which uses the argon laser to focus light on the retina in the back of the eye through the dilated pupil. When the laser light hits vessels on the surface of the retina, the light is transferred into heat energy. When reacting with the protein tissue, the laser light causes coagulation, thus destroying microaneurisms, leaky vessels and new vessel formation, and other damaged or compromised microvascular conditions on the surface of the retina. It is well established that this therapy markedly decreases retinal hemorrhages and proliferation of vessels on and around the retina. The first form of photocoagulation did not utilize a laser as light source. In 1959, a high-pressure xenon arc bulb system was used as the first treatment modality for diabetic retinopathy, and thus the term *photocoagulation* was coined. The argon laser was first introduced in 1968, and over the years since its acceptance into the medical treatment protocol for diabetic retinopathy, it has been refined as a high-tech therapy. Interestingly, the blue-green light of the argon laser is well absorbed by the highly compromised and abnormal red vasculature on the retina of the diabetic with retinopathy. The laser light beam is a well-controlled, very manageable thin beam of light that is focused through a forty-power lens placed on the corneal surface of the eye. The ophthalmologist looks through this lens as he or she strikes the abnormal vessels with pinpoint accuracy. This coagulation accuracy goes down to the fifty-micrometer level and the time of exposure can be one-fiftieth of a second or longer, depending on the durability and size of the vessel involved. This procedure is painless and no anesthesia is required, except topical anesthetic eyedrops.

Should the complicated diabetic eye become even more complicated, a surgical procedure called vitrectomy can be performed. The procedure is medically termed *pars planar vitrectomy* and has been touted as a rather promising operation for diabetic eyes that are blind due to vitreous hemorrhage. The surgical device itself is approximately the size of a sixteen-gauge needle. This needle device is inserted into the central vitreous of the eye. It is a combination device that has a cutting needle and both ingoing infusion and outgoing suction capability. The small motor drive is located on the handle of the instrument itself. In this way blood and tissue, including vascular membranes and fibrous bands, can be removed and replaced with a fresh, clear saline solution called Ringer's solution. This allows for a clear transmission of light to pass through the vitreous humor and back to the retina. The most successful vitrectomy cases have proven to be where the blindness is due primarily to hemorrhage into the vitreous humor and where membranes and fibrous tissue banding prevent light images from being picked up by the retina. A diabetic whose eye is too greatly damaged from advanced retinopathy, fibrosis, and degeneration would not be a candidate for this surgery.

What I have presented to you is the current understanding of the nature of diabetic eye disease. If we understood all the parameters involved, we could certainly prevent even more visual impairment and blindness due to diabetes. The harsh reality of even the most remote possibility of losing eyesight or going totally blind from diabetes is one of the most traumatizing emotional events experienced by those of us with diabetes.

Remember that knowledge is strength. The more you know about diabetes, the better your life will be. Because you are aware of the problems you may or may not encounter does not mean that you will definitely experience these situations just because you are well informed. I think this is an important concept for you to ponder over and get comfortable with as you live your life with diabetes. When I meet another diabetic who has had the disease for fewer years than I, it is only normal for that diabetic to become emotionally involved when he or she discovers that the cause of my total blindness is due to the very disease that afflicts us both.

What is the future for diabetic eye disease? There is tremendous hope within the pharmaceutical industry that major advances will be made through the use of rather elegant drug therapy. Experts feel that the state of the art for laser therapy and microsurgical vitrectomy is at hand. These techniques have been perfected through years and years of clinical practice. New instrumentation and refinement of lighting in the surgical field within the eye has greatly improved the vitrectomy surgical procedure.

The two newest avenues for the reduction of diabetic eye disease are aldose reductase inhibitors and amino guanidine. These new drug therapies are on the near frontier for the future of better control of severe diabetic complications. Merrill Dow has taken a leadership role in the formulation of these drugs, designed to retard or prevent diabetic retinopathy. Clinical trials with these new agents are under way, and hopefully we will soon see a time when this complication of long-term diabetes can be completely eliminated.

Joan Miller, Anthony Adamis, and ten other ophthalmology researchers at the Massachusetts Eye and Ear Infirmary, Children's Hospital, and Beth Israel Hospital, in Boston have discovered a protein that stimulates the abnormal growth of the small blood vessels emanating from the retina of diabetic animals. Their work is based on thirty years of research into proliferative blood-vessel growth conducted by Dr. Judith Holkman at Children's Hospital. This discovery is so important that it may mean the difference between sight and blindness for many thousands of people affected by diabetes and other retinal diseases distinguished by a proliferation of the tiny blood vessels in the back of the eye.

A hormonelike protein called vascular endothelial growth factor (VEGF) is believed to correlate closely with the extent of damage from diabetic retinopathy in monkeys. This correlation suggests that VEGF is responsible for the abnormal growth of blood vessels.

The team of ophthalmologists believes that the growth may be stopped and the retina saved. There are several drugs undergoing extensive research at this time that may be able to block this growth factor and thus prevent diabetic retinopathy and loss of sight.

Studies of human diabetic patients with and without retinopathy as compared to nondiabetics indicate that VEGF is significantly elevated in patients with diabetic retinopathy. Experiments to confirm the preliminary results are hoped to help find treatments that will block VEGF production.

This is exciting news for the millions of diabetics who have not suffered diabetic retinopathy and for those who are destined to become diabetics in the future. Slowly, the pieces of this incredible puzzle within an enigma are being put together. Certainly, it will take some time before the results of experimental data can provide useful treatments at the patient level. However, we will all rejoice when the long-awaited day comes that brings an end to diabetic retinopathy.

The newly diagnosed diabetic must learn discipline from the outset. By learning to control your blood sugar to well within the normal range, the dread complication of diabetic retinopathy may be prevented entirely, or at least minimized. Make up your mind right now that this complication is not going to destroy your life and that you are going to do all that is humanly possible to prevent it. Does this mean that you should live only for your diabetes and give up everything that is enjoyable in life? No, but I do think that if you work diligently over the long term toward maintaining normalized blood sugars, your chances of preventing this complication are better than the chances of the diabetic who does little in terms of taking care of his diabetes.

Obviously, diminished vision and blindness constitute the major fear of all diabetics and is certainly recognized by our federal government as a severe handicap. Less than 1 percent of new blindness was associated with diabetes in 1930. In 1960, this figure had risen to over 15 percent, and by 1980, over 23 percent of cases of new blindness in the United States were due to diabetic retinopathy. Diabetes is the most clinically significant systemic condition causing blindness in all age groups. There are literally tens of thousands of diabetics who have become totally blind or visually impaired due to long-term diabetes. We are no longer members of an exclusive club, and a renewed effort should be undertaken within the research community to find better ways to prevent the tragedy of blindness for the diabetic. I would like to remind you that just because you are diabetic and live long enough with this disease to be called long-term, that does not mean that you will become blind, or even suffer any damage to your vision at all. It seems as though some diabetics are genetically predisposed to vascular complications that involve the eye and some are not.

If you should be diagnosed with diabetic retinopathy, you must get beyond fear and carefully work out a plan of action with your endocrinologist or internist and your ophthalmologist. I cannot emphasize this point enough: after the diagnosis of retinopathy, if your blood sugars are not under good control, then do something about it. If this means checking yourself into the hospital for a week or two in order to get the help you need, then by all means do it. Your stress level will tend to interfere with your good blood glucose control and it will require even more discipline and perhaps additional insulin to get your diabetes under control. This aspect is extremely important and one that must be scrupulously followed if laser treatments are to be given the chance to prevent loss of vision.

What else can one do in fighting the progressive nature of this disease? Positive visualization and use of positive mind-sets may indeed be the future for better health. The use of the mind to heal the body is not a new thought. Aristotle and Hippocrates both postulated that the mind heals the body. One must consider whether it is more desirable to remain negative, bitter, frustrated, and projecting degeneration and illness for one's future, or positive, happy, and projecting only the best health condition for one's future through positive mental visualization. One must see clearly the visual image of total health. Even if this ideal state is not achieved, certainly one will feel better no matter what the future holds. Think about this and try it in your own life.

9

Long-term Complications to the Diabetic Kidney

Renal insufficiency, or kidney disease and failure, is the largest cause of death in the diabetic population in those who are diagnosed with this disease before age twenty. When one stops to think about this fact, the devastation of diabetes begins to wield its full impact. Diabetic kidney disease, known as diabetic nephropathy, is the chronic presence of protein in the urine, termed proteinuria, in the long-term diabetic, and is further defined as nephropathy without any other kidney disease present. It is interesting to note that the diabetic kidney undergoes many functional and morphological changes before the clinical diagnosis of diabetic nephropathy is determined. Most experts agree that in Type I insulin-dependent diabetes, diabetic nephropathy follows a well-defined and predictable course from onset of constant proteinuria to renal insufficiency, end-stage renal disease, or death.

In Type I diabetes, constant proteinuria may develop after fourteen to nineteen years with diabetes, with severe kidney insufficiency developing within four to five years later and end-stage renal disease or death following within a year, unless suitable hemodialysis or renal transplantation is performed. In Type II diabetes, proteinuria occurs earlier after the clinical diagnosis of diabetes is made, but often does not bring with it the severe renal insufficiency found in Type I diabetes.

After fifteen years of diabetes, approximately 33 percent of those with Type I diabetes and 20 percent of those with Type II diabetes will develop diabetic nephropathy. Factors associated with a higher incidence of diabetic nephropathy within the diabetic population are hypertension, poor blood sugar control, and smoking.

Fortunately, today we have several defenses to fight against these factors. First, we have better antihypertensive medication to combat high blood pressure and its devastating effects on the diabetic (see Chapter 11 on hypertension page 72). Second, we have improved blood glucose control due to self home blood glucose monitoring. The results of the Diabetes Control and Complications Trial show that tight blood glucose control helps in preventing diabetic nephropathy and its untoward effects. Finally, we now all know the absurdities of smoking in the light of the prolific amount of scientific data revealing the damage smoking can cause by increasing blood pressure and thereby endangering the kidneys.

There is one basic difference between the eye and the kidney as target organs for diabetic complications: you can live without your eyesight, but you cannot live without your kidneys. The kidneys are absolutely vital in filtering out nitrogenous waste products from the blood; should the kidneys fail to perform, without immediate medical attention death will ensue.

For the average person, the kidneys are about the size of your clenched fist. Inside each kidney is an absolute wonderment of intricately specialized structures and microvasculature involving incredibly complex biochemical and physiological function. We tend to take these organs for granted when they are performing correctly. However, once you study their form and function, I do not think you will take them for granted ever again.

The kidneys are located to the rear of the abdominal cavity and are just in back of the peritoneum, imbedded in a considerable amount of fat. In the adult male, each kidney weighs about 125 to 175 grams (approximately 4 to 6 ounces). Because the liver is present on the right side of the body, the right kidney is approximately two to eight centimeters (one to two inches) lower than the left kidney.

Each kidney, structurally, is surrounded by a discrete layer of fascia, a sheet of fibrous tissue that splits into two leaflets, one in front and one in back of each kidney. Above and to the side of each kidney, the leaflets fuse together, thereby partially enclosing each kidney with its associated adrenal gland. Unique layers of fat keep the kidneys in position and allow them some motility when a person changes position from supine to erect.

Each kidney is enclosed in a fibrous capsule, called the renal capsule. The purpose of the renal capsule is to provide a barrier against the spread of infection. The inside cavity of the kidney is called the renal sinus, and this cavity opens at the midpoint. It is at this midpoint that additional structures enter into the kidney. The renal artery enters into the kidney at this point and branches extensively, thus supplying blood to renal segments. It is also at this midpoint that the renal vein leaves the kidney.

The kidney is further divided into two parts. The cortex contains renal corpuscles, proximal convoluted tubules, renal columns of Bertini, and distal convoluted tubules. The medulla is composed of straight tubules, Henle's loops, and collecting ducts.

The kidney is further subdivided into lobes. Each renal pyramid, with the overlying cortex and adjacent regions of renal columns, forms the basic component of the kidney, the lobe. Pyramids are fusions of lobes.

Functionally, it is vitally important that the kidneys preserve minerals and help to establish electrolyte balance within the body fluids. It is this delicate balance that is so disturbed in undiagnosed or uncontrolled diabetes and in diabetic ketoacidosis.

Inside each kidney are ten million or more nephrons (from nephros, meaning kidney). Each nephron, the functional unit of the kidney, is composed of the renal corpuscle, the proximal convoluted tubule, the nephronic loop, and the distal convoluted tubule.

The ultrafiltrate of plasma, a component of blood, is called provisional urine. This provisional urine proceeds on to the glomerular capillaries and then into Bowman's capsule, which is the beginning of the nephron. Along the proximal tubule, specific substances are absorbed from provisional urine, and this results in the osmotic uptake of water, while other substances are secreted into the provisional urine by the tubules. It is in the distal tubule that sodium and water may or may not be absorbed, depending on the concentration of two specific hormones, antidiuretic hormone and aldosterone. Thus, the fluid that remains passes on to the collecting ducts and is excreted as urine. In the normal adult, approximately one hundred fifty to two hundred liters of provisional urine are produced each day, while reabsorption results in the production of about one to two liters of urine.

It was first noted in the 1930s that the basement membranes of long-term diabetics were thickened abnormally in the glomerular structures found within the kidneys (see Chapter 10, page 68, and the discussion on diabetic angiopathy). This led to discovery of further organ involvement in the micro- and macroangiopathy disease process in the long-term diabetic.

The first sign of diabetic nephropathy is intermittent glomerular proteinuria. Normal or above-normal glomerular filtration rates continue as protein excretion is continuous, and the amount of protein excretion increases. Thereafter, glomerular filtration rate falls and further renal function deteriorates. When other causes of proteinuria are absent (heart failure, urinary tract infection), this condition in diabetics is almost always due to diabetic renal microvascular disease. Primarily, this kidney disease is due to glomerulopathy, or the deterioration of blood vessels around the glomerulus. The thickening of the basement membrane within the glomerulus of the kidney is the prime cause of the ultimate failure of this organ system. Diabetics are also prone to other disease states of the kidney, including hardening of the large arteries that bring the kidneys their blood supply.

In terms of kidney function, the important aspect to look at is the glomerular filtration rate. This is a numerical value assigned to the actual filtration rate performed by the glomerular structures within the kidney. It is now thought to be the basement membrane thickening that gradually and progressively, over the long term, occludes the opening of the glomerulus and thus reduces the glomerular surface area and the glomerular filtration rate. It has been estimated that by the time the diabetic has fifteen years' experience with diabetes, especially in the type I insulin-dependent diabetic, over 50 percent of the glomerular structures are occluded and thus nonfunctioning. With time, renal insufficiency develops to the point that the organ is no longer functional at all. If the remaining kidney becomes nonfunctional, the diabetic is forced to undergo kidney dialysis and begin the waiting process for a suitable donor replacement organ.

One type of dialysis is hemodialysis. With this method, a simple surgical procedure is first performed to create a fistula in the forearm. This provides the entryway for the dialysis tubing. This fistula is kept clean and is washed with heparin, which removes any clotted blood. A team-management approach is necessary here for the best results. The internist or endocrinologist, the nephrologist or kidney specialist, the dialysis nurse, and the diabetic must all work together for the best results.

Each dialysis treatment may last five hours or more, depending on body weight and other factors, and may be required three or four times per week. Blood urea nitrogen (BUN) and creatinine clearance are carefully monitored to calculate how well the blood is being cleaned. Blood glucose testing is also done to make sure the levels are not too high or too low. Some diabetics still urinate, indicating there may be some remaining kidney function. This is usually not sufficient to properly rid the body of waste, but it may mean dialysis can be done less frequently.

Fortunately, today there are several new types of dialysis available that allow a great deal of freedom. However, their success still depends on following detailed instructions. One procedure uses a relatively new type of dialysis called continuous ambulatory peritoneal dialysis (CAPD). It is a home therapy in which the patient's peritoneal sac (a membrane that lines the abdominal cavity) is used to remove waste products and extra fluid from the body. An indwelling catheter is surgically placed through the abdominal wall, and dialysis solution is allowed to flow into the body through the catheter. The solution remains inside the peritoneum for four to eight hours while the patient goes about his or her daily routine. Waste products and extra fluid then flow out through the catheter. Fresh dialysis solution is prepared and infused after each four- to eight-hour period. This is continued three to four times daily.

Continuous ambulatory peritoneal dialysis requires special training in order to carry the procedure out correctly. Meticulous cleanliness and sterile technique must be followed for this type of dialysis and there are special ultraviolet light exchange tools you must learn to use to prevent bacteria from entering the peritoneum. Should bacteria enter the peritoneal cavity, serious infection could occur because the peritoneum is a sterile cavity with no white blood cells to fight infections.

With patient and exacting attention to detail, it is possible for most diabetics, sighted or not, to be able to use this technique. Special adaptive aids are available for people with visual impairments. However, loss of sensation in the fingers can be a problem with CAPD. One of the benefits to this type of dialysis is that insulin is given directly into the indwelling catheter, so injections might no longer be necessary. In my opinion, it is best if you have a partner trained to assist with this type of dialysis. Discuss the pros and cons of any type of dialysis with your doctor.

A new type of peritoneal dialysis, called continuous cycling peritoneal dialysis (CCPD), is becoming more popular. This type of dialysis is done at night while the patient is asleep, freeing the daytime for normal activities.

Diabetics who have been determined to have advanced kidney failure are diagnosed with end-stage renal disease, ESRD. If this condition goes untreated, then uremia (a condition of excess nitrogenous wastes in the blood) and death may soon follow. In 1990, the cost of treating ESRD, for all patients with ESRD including the diabetic population in the United States, amounted to more than $7 billion.

Ever since statistics have been kept for this disease, the incidence and prevalence rates of ESRD treatment have increased without showing signs of letting up. The age-, race-, and gender-adjusted incidence rate of ESRD treatment increased by 7.8 percent per year between 1985–1987 and 1988–1990. By 1990, the number of patients treated for ESRD amounted to two hundred ten thousand annually. Current projections predict the number may be close to three hundred thousand by the year 2000.

Diabetes may account for up to 33 percent of all cases of ESRD in the United States. The risk of ESRD is much greater with Type I diabetes than Type II. Although there is a greater preponderance of Type II diabetes, about 80 percent of the fourteen to fifteen million diagnosed cases of diabetes, Type I diabetes still accounts for about 66 percent of all causes of diabetic ESRD.

A ten-year trial from the National Institutes of Health–supported Diabetes Control and Complications Trial, DCCT, suggests that strict control of blood sugar levels in Type I diabetes cuts in half the subsequent incidence of renal insufficiency. A larger ongoing multicenter treatment trial in Type II diabetics and a multicenter primary prevention of diabetes trial are being supported by the National Institutes of Health. Hopefully, this new data will help medical researchers and physicians to further decrease the incidence of diabetic nephropathy, renal insufficiency, and ESRD.

10

Long-term Complications to the Diabetic Vascular and Nervous Systems

The complication to the blood vessels of the diabetic known as diabetic microangiopathy is, like many other areas within the field of diabetes, not completely understood. A tremendous amount of medical research has been carried out in this area; however, most informative books on diabetes for the average reader do not include an explanation of this particular complication. If you understand this progressive state of micro–blood vessel disease, then you will better understand the major diabetic complications of diabetic kidney disease and eye disease.

To get oxygen to the tissues is the job of our exceedingly complex circulatory system, consisting of blood vessels and blood. It is also the responsibility of the circulatory system to remove products of metabolism and to deliver glucose and other energy-rich materials. Blood flows due to a pressure gradient that is maintained, and in order to deliver oxygen to all the tissues, an appropriate flow rate of the blood is required throughout the vascular system. The blood flow rate and the problems encountered as this flow surges through the blood vessel walls is a special study in fluid mechanics. The study of blood flow within the vascular system and the delivery of oxygen to tissues is important here because of the myriad changes that occur over the long term within the diabetic.

Medically, the word *angiopathy* means any disease of the blood vessels. We are discussing diabetic angiopathy, in particular the angiopathy that affects the microvasculature, although diabetic macroangiopathy affects the larger blood vessels. In order to picture the level with which we are dealing, we must understand the overall vascular system itself. First there are the major arteries and veins that progressively branch and differentiate into the smaller arteries and veins, then the very small arteries and veins called arterioles and venules, then the capillary beds and microvessels, and finally the microscopic and submicroscopic vessels within this most intricate system of blood flow. The study of blood in all aspects from anatomy to pathology is a medical specialty called hematology. The study of the vascular system and the dynamics of blood in the diabetic is a critically important area within diabetes due to the complications experienced during the lifetime of the diabetic.

In 1936 it was discovered that vascular abnormalities existed within the delicate structures of the kidneys of diabetic patients. Later, it was found that these abnormalities were also present in other organs of the diabetics who had had the disease for many years. By the 1950s, a sufficient number of diabetics had survived with diabetes over the long term to make studies of these abnormalities possible. It was during this time that vascular specialists were beginning to understand that diabetes involves a very distinct set of complications to the blood vessels of the human body, and the term *microangiopathy* was coined to describe this condition.

With the development of the electron microscope, it was found that the small blood vessels in long-term diabetics had a common factor, a thickening of the basement membrane found inside the blood vessel wall that took place gradually, over a number of years. The term *basement membrane* was first used by histologists, those who study the microanatomy of the cellular structures of cells, tissues, and organs in relation to their functions. The basement membrane is a bandlike structure beneath the basal surface of various skin layers; the term has been widened to include basement membranous structures of varying degrees of thickness, location, and dimension. Basement membrane thickening was a very important finding in the research of diabetes. It is important that you understand the progressive nature of this thickening, since it ultimately leads to the deleterious clinical complications found in long-term diabetes.

The degradation of nerve pathways of the diabetic, known as diabetic neuropathy, is not a condition limited to the diabetic, but it is probably the most common diabetic complication, even though it is still poorly understood. It involves the diabetic's total body, places all systems at risk, and plays a significant role in many other areas of diabetes including hormonal secretory mechanisms and regulation, visceral functions, and many other nonneurologic complications within the diabetic state.

It is the current opinion of research endocrinologists, and others studying diabetic complications, that the underlying mechanism of diabetic neuropathy is of a multisyndrome effect divided into categories whose cause is either vascular or metabolic, or a combination of the two. At the microscopic level, it is thought that neuropathy causes segmental demyelination of the peripheral nerve fibers. This means that the protective nerve covering called myelin is somehow broken down and stripped off the nerve fibers in a segmental fashion. Spirally folded Schwann cells form the myelin sheath, and it is further thought that the metabolism of the Schwann cell is somehow interfered with during the process of diabetic neuropathy.

The Schwann cell is responsible for the elaboration of myelin and is believed to play an important part in the energy metabolism of the nerve axon. Research into the involvement of the Schwann cell has indicated that its role in diabetic neuropathy is evident since damage to these cells results in demyelination, remyelination, and segmental loss of myelin of single-fiber peripheral nerve cells obtained from patients with a long history of diabetic neuropathy. It is now the opinion of many researchers that it is the nerve axon itself that degenerates in both peripheral and sympathetic nerves of diabetics; furthermore, this degeneration favors the unmyelinated nerve fibers.

Diabetic peripheral neuropathy is a painful condition usually associated with the extremities, namely the lower legs. The pain can manifest itself as a burning sensation or sharp pain that is so acute it will wake up the diabetic in the middle of the night, the time when neuropathy is usually more acute. Diabetic neuropathy is a complication encountered in longer-term diabetes, mostly after several years of uncontrolled high blood glucose. Sugar proteins, called glycoproteins, form in the nerves after some years with uncontrolled high blood glucose. For some reason, this deposition of glycoprotein occurs primarily in the nerves of the lower extremities; however, neuropathy can occur elsewhere in the diabetic. Severe neuropathy is an aggravation and there is not a lot that can be done to alleviate it.

Capsaicin, an extract from hot peppers that gives them their fiery taste, is a new hope for diabetics who experience painful peripheral neuropathy. This drug is found naturally in the peppers that are used to make Tabasco sauce and some salsas, a traditional dish of spices, peppers, and other ingredients often combined in a tomato base. I eat a lot of salsa and I find that the natural capsaicin in the peppers has reduced my neuropathy to zero. I have not suffered any neuropathy pain in years, and salsa is always part of my lunch. Capsaicin can now be purchased at health-food stores and pharmacies. Ask your doctor; there should be no problem in taking it to help prevent neuropathy because this is a safe, naturally occurring product.

Some of the older physicians who treat long-term diabetics have reported that vitamin B12 injections (sometimes in conjunction with thiamine) have alleviated some painful diabetic neuropathy. Ask your doctor what he does in the treatment of neuropathy.

11

Implications of Hypertension for the Diabetic

When I was in my late teens and early twenties, one of the last things I worried about, in terms of my health, was high blood pressure, or hypertension. Our level of understanding of high-blood-pressure control and the ability to manage a patient with this condition was abysmally poor at that time. In the thirty-two years since I was diagnosed with diabetes, there have been miraculous medical advances. A partial list includes heart transplant surgery pioneered by Dr. Christian Barnard in the early seventies, the life-saving techniques of saphenous vein coronary artery bypass graft surgery developed by Drs. Michael DeBakey and Denton Cooley in the early 1970s, the advent of self home blood glucose monitors in the mid '70s, and the new use of imaging techniques in the early '80s.

Tremendous advances have been made in the field of pharmacology, with the pharmaceutical industry developing today's new antidiabetic oral medications, new antianxiety agents to relieve the stress of high anxiety and depression, new techniques of wound healing, and new drugs to promote the better functioning of the heart and to reduce high blood pressure. We are fortunate to live in an age of high technology and advancement into the new millennium with doctors, researchers, and scientists dedicating their lives and devoting many long, hard hours to provide an enlightened and improved hope for the future and our better health.

On the average, the diabetic will suffer more from all forms of heart disease and malfunction than his nondiabetic counterpart. These conditions include myocardial infarction, coronary artery disease, angina pectoris, and congestive heart failure.

Atherosclerosis is a disease that begins early in life. It has been determined by the International Atherosclerosis Project that by ages ten to fourteen, fatty streaks within the aorta are already significant for up to 20 percent of blacks and 5 to 6 percent of whites. Fibrous plaques are found to be common by the third decade of life. It is no wonder that today doctors and scientists are constantly urging young people to watch their intake of fatty foods. Prevention of cardiovascular disease in young people is scientifically justified. Certainly, one can see that should a young person develop diabetes, and, furthermore, should that young person be developing early atherosclerosis, the combination will add a tremendous burden to his heart and vascular system. Today young people tend to eat large quantities of fatty junk foods and to participate less and less in vigorous outdoor sports and activities; the diabetic must work even harder to overcome these alarming statistics.

It has been estimated that the prevalence of coronary artery disease is 1.2 to 6.6 times greater for the diabetic population than for their nondiabetic counterparts. Indeed, diabetics are prone to an increased incidence of fatty streaks, atherosclerotic lesions, fibrous plaques, calcified lesions, and coronary stenosis, all of which are complications to the coronary arteries. Generally, the prevalence of coronary artery disease seems to increase with the duration of diabetes but does not correlate with the severity of diabetes. It has been reported that coronary artery disease is the most common cause of death in the Type II diabetic, but it is commonly found in the Type I diabetic as well.

The influence of the effects of diabetes is much greater for peripheral vascular disease (disease of the arteries and veins of the legs and feet) than it is for coronary heart disease. If, on the other hand, other risk factors are present, including hyperlipidemia (high blood fat levels), hypercholesterolemia (high cholesterol levels), increased age, hypertension, and electrocardiogram (ECG) evidence of left ventricular hypertrophy, the impact of diabetes is greater on coronary heart disease. It is important to note that even when these risk factors are taken into account, the influence of diabetes on coronary disease is still present.

The angiotensin-converting enzyme inhibitors, known as ACE inhibitors, are an important pharmacologic tool that enables the diabetic to control his hypertension. It is crucial to your better understanding of diabetes that you realize the importance of controlling high blood pressure. The diabetic's system is placed on overload when the heart becomes compromised and thus must work harder and harder to pump blood to all parts of the body. It has long been an important theory within diabetes research that one of the most serious problems in the diabetic's body is not only getting blood to all parts of the tissues, but providing enough oxygen to keep these tissues alive and performing properly. By reducing the load on the heart and the strain on the vascular system, organs such as the eyes and kidneys, which are directly and indirectly affected by long-term diabetes, could have their lifetime extended by reducing hypertension. Researchers have long been aware of the added complications hypertension can cause, not only in the diabetic population, but in the nondiabetic population as well. Imagine for just a moment the tremendous additional burden the diabetic must undergo when told his eyes and kidneys are suffering from long-term effects of diabetes. Immediately, the stress level is increased almost intolerably, along with hypertension and emotional overload. Adequate steps must be undertaken to help relieve this stressful situation, and close consultation with your medical team is essential.

The future looks promising for the reduction of hypertension and damage to the eyes and kidneys, heart and vascular system of the diabetic, due to the ACE inhibitor captopril (trade name Capoten, made by Bristol-Myers Squibb). The medical indications for use of this enzyme inhibitor is rapidly expanding and, as an added bonus, it is known to make the patient feel better. In 1986, a quality-of-life study was undertaken by Sidney H. Croog and colleagues that showed that captopril gave a much better quality of life than other agents when used in the treatment of hypertension. Researchers found that when captopril was used, important aspects of life such as social behavior, sexual function, and intellectual performance were maintained at a high level. This is due to the far-reaching implications of angiotensin II, a potent vasoconstrictor that is a powerful stimulus for the production and release of aldosterone. Aldosterone is a steroid hormone produced by the adrenal cortex, and its major action is to facilitate potassium exchange for sodium in the distal renal tubule. This action causes sodium reabsorption and potassium and hydrogen loss. All of these vital biochemical steps are important regulatory functions required to maintain life.

During the renin-angiotensin cycle, when blood flow is restricted to the kidneys, a peptide called renin is secreted. When renin is secreted by the kidneys, it converts circulating angiotensinogen to angiotensin I. The angiotensin-converting enzyme converts angiotensin I to angiotensin II, which is a powerful blood vessel constrictor, or vasoconstrictor. Constriction of the very small blood vessels in the peripheral parts of the body, called peripheral arterioles, produces increased blood pressure and therefore increased blood flow to the kidneys. This process, known as the renin-angiotensin system, is now well understood within the discipline of biochemistry.

Captopril was the first drug to be "designed," that is, its development was based on its molecular interaction with a specific target. It was released as an antihypertensive. A brilliant research team, headed by Leonard T. Skeggs at the VA Hospital and Western Reserve University in Cleveland, Ohio, were responsible for separating the two forms of circulating angiotensin in 1954. Clinicians were advised that this drug must be used with great caution due to possible side effects, which include an allergic-type rash, fever, proteinuria, or leukopenia. These side effects are not seen as much today due to the fact that the dosage levels have been brought down to around 125 mg/day or less instead of earlier dosages of three to ten times higher.

From the use of captopril, I have experienced a chronic cough, one of the more recently reported effects seen with this drug. Although the cough is bothersome, the benefits greatly outweigh the side effect, since the drug allows maintaining good blood pressure control and preserving my kidney function. Fortunately, ACE inhibitors have proved to be not only simple to use, but also among the safest of the cardiac drugs. There are seventeen different ACE inhibitors on the market around the world, seven of which are available in the United States. There are no indications at this time that one ACE inhibitor is superior to another; however, your doctor may have a preference due to your particular medical history.

Captopril has proved to be beneficial for the insulin-dependent diabetic. Studies have shown that it has lowered the number of deaths of insulin-dependent diabetics with renal disease and has decreased the number of patients who have had to have renal transplants or undergo hemodialysis. At first, researchers were puzzled as to why this was happening and thought that perhaps it was due to the reduction in hypertension. However, it is now thought that a renal protective process is at work with captopril. The mechanism of this process is still under intense study, but the present reasoning is that ACE inhibitors lessen the blood pressure in the renal arterioles; this causes an unloading of minute glomerular capillaries where filtration of urine occurs. It is these minute glomerular capillaries that the degradation process of diabetes attacks.

Captopril may also be useful to the non-insulin-dependent diabetic. It is insulin resistance that is of concern to the Type II diabetic, and it is hoped that captopril may reduce this problem. Insulin resistance occurs, to our best knowledge, when, during the glucose fatty acid cycle, the fatty acid inhibits the utilization of glucose. Then, more insulin is required to get the glucose into the cell, with the result that the insulin concentration rises in the blood. In both the obese and the hypertensive patient, insulin falls short in the promotion of the uptake of glucose. At the present time, there seems to be no real explanation for insulin resistance. Researchers at Stanford University School of Medicine believe that insulin resistance may be a metabolic defect that explains why many obese patients may have the tendency to develop hypertension, diabetes, or both.

Dr. John Raia at Bristol-Myers Squibb Pharmaceutical says that Capoten is now limited to the treatment of diabetic nephropathy with proteinuria of 500 mg/day in patients with Type I insulin-dependent diabetes mellitus and retinopathy in patients with or without hypertension. Capoten has been found to be safe and effective in decreasing the rate of progression of renal insufficiency, which can lead to dialysis, the need for renal transplantation, or death. Capoten is also indicated in the treatment of hypertension, congestive heart failure, and left ventricular dysfunction after myocardial infarction. This new indication for captopril is based on a study published in the *New England Journal of Medicine* by Lewis and colleagues (1993). Captopril was shown to significantly reduce the risk of morbidity and mortality associated with end-stage renal disease, ESRD, for diabetic patients. Captopril is the first ACE inhibitor to demonstrate efficacy in improving clinical outcomes in patients with diabetic nephropathy, including reduced risk for necessary dialysis therapy and renal transplantation.

Six years ago an internal medicine specialist recommended that I be placed on a daily intake of up to 150 mg Capoten as an antihypertensive agent in addition to a diuretic, furosemide, trade name Lasix. As a result, my blood pressure control is good and my kidneys, even though I do show some protein spillage into my urine as measured on a twenty-four-hour urine collection, are still in quite good shape.

I believe that it would be in your best interest to monitor your blood pressure and consult with your doctor on the advisability of adding captopril to your medical armamentarium if appropriate. Although Bristol-Myers Squibb cannot advise a prophylactic use of captopril if you are not showing any signs of hypertension or nephropathy, consult with your doctor and make sure you take any sign of high blood pressure seriously. We are, indeed, fortunate today to have modern, high-technology pharmacology working with us to help us deal with the more insidious aspects of diabetes.

12

Taking a Positive Approach

There was a time in my sighted life when I greatly desired to go racing. I have always had a great passion for cars, so why not push it to the limit and race Ferraris for sport? I had some lengthy discussions with an experienced Ferrari man, representatives from the Ferrari distributor, and some wealthy financial backers who were also interested in the cars and racing. We discussed obtaining a Ferrari 512 Berlinetta Boxer LM, fully race-prepared for LeMans, from the factory. We would obtain an enclosed trailer and a full-time mechanic, and enter the GT race circuit.

All of this sounded great to me, because I wanted to do the driving. Then the discussion turned to "what ifs." What if the car is wrecked—should we have a spare? What if the driver is injured? What if the entire program becomes too expensive? The discussion got so negative and paranoid that we even got to the point of asking: What if, during a race, the tire pressure gauge is affected by different weather and barometric conditions, throwing off our tire pressures? After a while, we asked: What if we just had not started this discussion in the first place?

I am sure that most of us go through many different scenarios of "what ifs," and I do believe that preparing one's mind for possible future problems is not all bad. However, it is also my opinion that setting the most positive reference points with positive attitudinal thinking is the best way to go. This allows the brain to set up positive mental images rather than the negative ones that can do us so much harm.

Certainly, this is part of the visualization techniques needed to help in your dealing with diabetes on a daily basis. There really are no limitations when it comes to the power of the mind.

When initially diagnosed with diabetes, either insulin-dependent or not, the mind starts asking "what ifs." As in my racing discussion above, doing this can result in creating giant mental obstacles that may or may not even exist.

Today, the number-one fear for most Americans is cancer, with blindness close behind. Why do we have this fear of losing our eyesight? The answer is obvious. We depend upon our sight more than any other sense. With tens of thousands of newly diagnosed diabetics having to deal with this disease every year, it is no wonder that the fear of diabetes and its many implications may cause us to ask, "What if I should begin to have eyesight problems or lose my eyesight entirely?"

By telling you my own story dealing with impending blindness, perhaps I can communicate to you the incredible mental anguish I underwent and how it required all my strength just to survive. Please read this with the understanding that eye research, laser technology, and retinal surgery have advanced ten years since the early 1980s. Although diabetes remains the number-one cause of new blindness in the United States, it is my hope that this situation becomes reversible through the efforts of new pharmacologic therapy, improved laser and surgical techniques, and further refinements in maintaining normalized blood glucose.

The experience of losing one's eyesight is devastating. One's lifestyle, whatever it may be, must be changed. It is a change that is all-encompassing, a mind-set that, in total, must be adapted to fall within new parameters. No matter what age you lose your sight after age six, when the visual cortex has developed sufficiently to create visual memory, it is a shocking revolt to the body's perceptual reflexes.

I was diagnosed with diabetes mellitus at age fifteen. Two different doctors missed the initial diagnosis two years earlier. I had the typical symptoms of uncontrolled diabetes, including extreme thirst, frequent urination, weight loss, listlessness, and malaise, a feeling of weakness. It was my wise grandmother and mother who noticed the fruity smell to my breath, the frequent urination, and the appearance of sticky patches around my bathroom toilet, like someone had spilled a sugar soft drink around the toilet area. This was due to the fact that I was spilling a tremendous amount of sugar into my blood, with the excess surpassing the renal threshold and being carried out through urination. With five or six trips to the bathroom in the middle of the night, it is no wonder that I would occasionally miss the toilet. This proved to be a blessing because, had I not begun insulin therapy soon, I most probably would have gone into a diabetic coma due to extreme hyperglycemia, or high blood sugar, and may not have survived.

The diagnosis of diabetes was accepted by me and I became compulsive in its ritual of shot-taking, boiling the glass syringes, and urine testing. I credit the diagnosis of diabetes with the impetus of leading me into the study of medicine. I was fully prepared to live with the daily insulin injections, urine testing, dietary restrictions, and increased healthful attitude the successful management of the disease required: thus, the making of a major lifestyle change at age fifteen.

During my early high-school years with diabetes, I pushed myself by getting up every morning at 4:30 A.M. to deliver the *Washington Post* newspaper. It was not only good discipline, but excellent exercise. As I became more experienced with my diabetes, I found I could do anything, from participating in the marching band to vigorous karate lessons. I was never the same after seeing Bruce Brown's wonderful 1966 surfing film, *Endless Summer*. I made up my mind to go to Hawaii to live, to go to college and surf the perfect waves that break on the reefs around the Hawaiian Islands. My sports were karate and surfing. Are these demanding sports appropriate for an individual with diabetes? I certainly thought they were and I earned a black belt in Japanese Shotokan karate, and I still train in the martial arts even today. I also became a big wave rider in the fantastic surf that breaks on the shallow reefs in the Hawaiian Islands. After my second year in Hawaii, I began surfing the big waves that break on Oahu's north shore. In the late 1960s we began riding short surfboards, approximately seven feet long. Before this time the average surfboard length was ten feet. The short boards required a tremendous amount of energy to paddle the one-quarter to one-half mile out to where the surf line began. The waves could be breaking at six to eight feet in height, then jump up to ten to fifteen feet in big sets. I controlled my diabetes exceedingly well to be able to survive the tremendous energy drain that surfing demands, and in four years, I never experienced an insulin reaction out in the surf. As I review my experiences surfing in the big waves off Oahu, I shudder to consider the "what ifs" that did not occur to me then.

There were many times that I surfed for five or six hours, then paddled to shore, all without suffering an insulin reaction. Just the mere thought of this today can frighten me, as I have endured enough insulin reactions to know quite well that an insulin reaction in thirty-foot waves could prove fatal. During my years in Hawaii, I knew of no other diabetics who surfed the big waves off Oahu's north shore. With today's intensified insulin therapy, a diabetic surfer who chooses to surf in the big waves should insure that adequate blood glucose levels are maintained before paddling out to the surf. Additionally, I would take along a waterproof pouch filled with honey or some other source of pure glucose so that if I were to become hypoglycemic, I could quickly squeeze the honey into my mouth while I began paddling to shore. Another good idea would be to surf with a buddy who is well aware of your diabetes and how to treat an insulin reaction.

After I graduated from college, I entered medical school. The heavy demands that reading, studying, and attending classes required were very difficult at times as a diabetic. Keeping up with the rest of the class was sometimes so difficult that I really wanted to give up. For convenience, mealtimes and shot times would have to be juggled, many times to the detriment of my diabetes, in order to work through whatever situation I was involved in at the medical school. There was test-taking almost every day, and the emotional stress along with the physical demands pushed me to the limits of my ability. But I made it through somehow, got married, and moved to California to do postgraduate medical research. I had become involved in basic clinical research of the molecular basis of diabetes while in medical school. The research was high-powered and demanding and required more than just a forty-hour week in order to be successful, so I gained insight into the emotional state of the working diabetic. Along with the work, I attained some financial success and became prone to the emotional stress and pressure that is required in order to maintain a successful lifestyle.

I was followed regularly by an endocrinologist or internist to provide objective management of my diabetes, and I paid meticulous attention to insulin injections, regular exercise, and a healthful diet, which included a lot of fresh vegetables and fruits. I therefore thought that I was doing everything I could do to control my disease.

In 1983, on a regular visit to my ophthalmologist, a retinal specialist and a friend who shared a mutual love of Ferraris and Porsche automobiles, my life changed in a few sentences.

"Joe, I hate like hell to tell you this," he said, swinging the slit lamp out of my way, "but you have a damn good case of retinopathy. We will have to begin laser treatments immediately. We will have two sessions a week, beginning with the right eye, which seems to be somewhat worse than the left."

He gave me no real choice. I knew the situation only too well. But this only happened to *other* diabetics, not me. I mean, why me? Why should this terrible condition happen to me? There are just too many things I have to accomplish in my life, and I am dependent on my eyesight to get these things done. After all, I rationalized, I am an artist who loves to oil paint and draw in black ink. I do meticulous medical research and like to drive fast sports cars. My life would be over were I to lose my eyesight.

Modern pan-retinal photocoagulation laser therapy was well known to save diabetics' vision. When I expressed the fear of going blind to my ophthalmologist friend, he told me how excellent my prognosis looked.

"Perhaps in seven or eight years we will have to do additional laser therapy, Joe, but we will be further along medically in understanding this condition," he said. "You have nothing to worry about. Your eyes are looking great."

But my eyes were not looking great. The intensity of the laser therapy knocked out my night vision, which had been excellent, after six months of treatments. Daily doses of vitamin A restored my night vision. I next developed vitreous floaters. These floaters are actually microparticles dislodged during the laser treatments. The particles float throughout the vitreous humor, the fluid-filled cavity in back of the lens. One Saturday, now in my eighth month of laser treatments, my wife and I went to our favorite restaurant. When the waitress brought the menus, I opened mine to look for my favorite dish. To my great surprise, I saw only a blank page. I asked my wife if I had been given a misprinted menu. Her shocked look told me everything. The menu was printed just fine; it was that I could not see it anymore. This was, of course, a gut-wrenching revelation. How was I going to continue my work at the medical school? My work demanded that my vision be critical and discerning in order to evaluate numerical data, color differentiations, and the myriad writing and tabulating of data and results to experiments, both basic research and clinical trials with patients. What was I going to do if I could not see fine print? I had the remainder of the weekend to ponder my dilemma.

On Monday morning, after I got to my office, my secretary brought me several phone messages and several letters I had written that required my signature. I studied the phone message sheet. I could make out the bold print, but not the handwriting of my secretary. Likewise, my letters appeared to be blank sheets, except for the bold medical school letterhead printed on the top. How would I tell everyone I need help? I decided to go to the nearest drugstore to purchase a pair of magnifying reading glasses. Maybe they would help me see the fine print. I had never worn glasses in all of my life. When I got back to my office, I put the glasses on and tried to read the phone messages. Holding them at arm's length, I could not see the handwriting. I placed the memo sheet at nose length and tried to read it. Just as I was beginning to read the numbers, my secretary walked in. She was horrified to see me with the memo sheet so close to my face. I brushed her off by saying that my eyesight had begun to change.

It certainly had begun to change, a critical change for the worse. I explained my fluctuating vision as due to my aggressive attempt to control my blood sugar. The stress at this time was unimaginable. Because my blood sugar was up and down, the lens, which is filled with a clear sugar solution called sorbitol, was being affected by the rise and fall in my blood sugar. This daily fluctuation affected my visual acuity from day to day. It was like being on a roller-coaster ride, one day up, the next down. My emotional state fluctuated in direct relationship to my visual performance.

The situation got worse. Every other day I worked out in a neighborhood park. The park had exercise stations with a set of equipment for sit-ups, push-ups, chin-ups, leg lifts, and so on, and a path for walking or jogging in-between stations. I was used to this training format and enjoyed it very much. I was now in the latter part of my eighth month of laser treatments. On this particular morning, about halfway through my exercise routine, I felt a fleeting sharp pain in my right eye. As I held one hand over my left eye in order to see the condition of the visual acuity in my right eye, I noticed a blurred patch in the upper left quadrant of my right eye. I had suffered my first major vitreous hemorrhage. This means that a blood vessel in the back of the right eye was starting to pump blood into the clear fluid between the retina, at the back of the eye, and the lens, at the front of the eye. I was almost panic-stricken. A vitreous hemorrhage is serious and threatens eyesight if not taken care of immediately. I called my ophthalmologist and got an appointment for the following day. Before I went in for the appointment, the left eye had also hemorrhaged. I could no longer see well enough to drive. I tried to drive to my office that morning and was just barely able to get back home without having an accident. I slid out from beneath the leather-wrapped steering wheel of my black Porsche 911 Turbo, never to drive it again. I did not fully realize it at the time, but I had just suffered one of the most devastating losses one can suffer, the loss of independence. It is truly hard to imagine the mental anguish one undergoes when the impact of the realization hits that, for the rest of your life, you will no longer be able to jump into your car and drive to wherever you want to go. The next time someone asks you to run an errand, like picking up a loaf of bread and some milk at the store, or when you are just taking a leisurely drive for the pleasure of it all by yourself, think about how it would be if you could no longer see to do these simple things.

My ophthalmologist told me what I already knew. Bilateral vitreous hemorrhages are quite serious. To my complete surprise, my proliferative retinopathy had turned into proliferative neovascularization, the burgeoning growth of new vessel formation, which leads directly to blindness. At this end stage of diabetic eye disease, a vitrectomy can be performed to save the eye as a last-ditch effort. A vitrectomy is a microsurgical operation. It involves the removal of the fluid within the vitreous humor, along with any weak vessels, and replacing the vitreous humor with clear saline. The entire operation is performed through an opening in the eye as large as a sixteen-gauge needle. The operation is extremely delicate, but there is a success rate of approximately 77 percent. I was referred to a retinal surgeon who performed vitrectomies. He evaluated me the following week. During that week, the retina in my right eye detached; I was now unable to see at all in that eye. The vitrectomy was to be performed in the left, good, eye. I entered the hospital able to see colors and make out shapes and forms. However, I could not see well enough to make out a person's face, even at close range. The surgery took three hours. There had been extensive tissue band growth due to the presence of fresh blood in the vitreous humor. The retinal surgeon had removed as much of the vessels and tissue as he could. I was experiencing allergic reactions to the anesthesia, so the decision was made to finish the surgery. Two thin threads of fibrin were left behind, attached to the top and bottom of the retina. After the surgery I was violently ill, a reaction to the anesthesia. And, of course, I had no vision. The left eye, which had just been operated on, had a patch on it. I was already blind in my right eye.

After several days in the hospital, I was released. We were all hoping that in a week's time, the blood would clear out of the vitreous humor and I would regain useful vision. My prognosis was for a return to at least 20/40 vision, good enough to read and drive. After six weeks I still could not see out of the left eye. I was weak and began experiencing extreme pain in the right temporal region of my head. The pain became so intense I felt as though I was having a burst in a cerebral aneurism. My head felt as though it were going to explode at any second. I was placed on narcotic analgesics and told the pain was due to a glaucoma complication. The painkillers, the strongest narcotics given, did little good in alleviating the tremendous pain. My glaucoma-affected right eye felt like a hard stone. The ocular pressure measured over 48. At this high internal ocular pressure, the pain is just barely tolerable. Eyes with this high a pressure have been known to literally burst. I was offered several options. An alcohol block could be administered into the optic nerve to stop the pain, cyclocryosurgery could be performed, or they could enucleate, remove, the eye.

I was now between a rock and a hard place. The decision was made by me to undergo the cyclocryotreatment in an effort to save the eye. In my situation, I was treated as an outpatient. A stainless-steel probe is cooled to -60°F with liquid nitrogen. The loop end of the probe is placed in a circular pattern around the eye. The probe is left on the surface of the eye for several minutes in each location as the circular pattern is completed. After the completion of this treatment I was taken home by my wife and was in acute pain for almost three hours. I was doing so poorly that my wife picked up the phone and called my parents. She was afraid I was going to die. So was I. It is difficult to put into words this intense pain. However, after several days, the pressure in the right eye subsided and the pain stopped. As a result of the trauma to the right eye, the left eye, which we had hoped would be returning to vision, became complicated. Just as some vision was beginning to return, the two fibrin strands that had been left attached to the retina began to stretch and pull on the retina. This meant that the retina was in danger of becoming detached. All of these complications were taking their toll. I lost forty pounds in six weeks. I was so weak that I could just barely muster the strength to walk. I had missed so much work that my job, indeed my career, was over. It was also during this emotionally troubling time that I discovered that my group medical insurance was denying payment to the hospital to cover my surgery. The reason? The surgery was deemed necessary because of a pre-existing condition, namely diabetes, that I had prior to obtaining my current group medical plan. Therefore, the payment was denied. My medical bills, even with some of it gratis, totaled about twenty-five thousand dollars at this point.

My wife could not deal with my intense suffering. I can fully understand this aspect now; I did not at the time. So, how do you feel when you are blind, out of a job, out of a career, deeply in debt, with no money coming in, and a spouse who wants a divorce in the middle of it all? Well, if you have the strength, you pray a lot. I know I certainly did. You must also count on those around you to help. My beloved mother and father were there to pick me up and nurture me back to health. It took some time. There were days that I could only tolerate living a minute at a time. When I had gathered up five minutes, I would go for another minute, and so on. The mental conditioning and challenge of my situation has changed me forever. No, my eyesight did not return, as I had hoped, prayed, and dreamed it would. On the other hand, I am still alive today, and indeed am quite healthy.

So, what is the message here? While we are on this earth, if we live long enough, each of us will be presented with the ultimate challenge. It may involve the death of a loved one, the loss of a limb or one of the five senses, or any multiplicity of life events that cause us to ask God, "Why me?" But, why not me? Terrible tragedies happen to people every hour of every day in real life. We really do have to take solace in our blessings. Life is fraught with challenge, and as in nature, only those who can meet the challenge and overcome adversity will survive.

With rehabilitation and the loving care of family and friends, I was able to meet the challenge. In fact, I meet it every day, because blindness does not go away. I am able to read magazines, books, and even medical journals through use of audiocassettes and flexible discs. I am able to get around by using a special white cane, and I am able to use a computer that enables me to gain access to information and write through the use of special artificial-intelligence voice synthesis. I am constantly amazed at what blind people can do. I once thought that life was over once you went blind. Now I know that life can still be great, and the only thing bad about being blind is that I cannot see.

Ultimately, every diabetic asks the questions, "Why do I have to have this dread disease, and why does diabetes produce such horrible complications?" These are very valid questions for which I have no real answer and ones that I myself have asked many times. With the development of modern medical techniques, the diabetic has been afforded a longer and longer life span. By living longer, the diabetic is now enduring the complications associated with long-term diabetes that he would not have had to endure before due to an early death.

Diabetes does not affect all who are living with this disease in the same manner. Not everyone with diabetes goes totally blind, nor do all diabetics lose kidney function and suffer bilateral leg amputations. It is true that diabetes is the number-one cause of new blindness within the United States, but many diabetics incur only the natural aging process associated with lens stiffening and thus require the usual remedy, that is, reading glasses or bifocals. Some diabetics will require treatment for retinopathy but may only require essential treatment that does not cause severe diminution of their vision. And of course many diabetics suffer kidney failure accompanying diabetic eye disease, making for a one-two punch that makes surviving extremely difficult. One can search for answers to the whys of all of this, but I have yet to find a satisfactory answer, and let me tell you, during my initial stage with total blindness, I had many solitary moments to contemplate diabetes in its entirety.

A diabetic acquaintance of mine can be an inspiration to you. Over nine years ago he lost his eyesight. He went into renal failure and was forced into kidney dialysis three to four times per week. After several years of kidney dialysis, a suitable transplant kidney was found, and although there were some initial setbacks, the transplanted kidney works well now. Over a year and a half ago, his right leg was amputated, but with diligent rehabilitation, he has learned to get around with a prosthetic replacement. Now he is facing permanent deafness due to nerve damage from the auditory canal to his brain. This sounds pretty grim, does it not? It would to this diabetic if he were not unique in his approach to life. His words are poignant and meaningful to those of us who have lost less: "I can see better with my totally blind eyes than those diabetics who are not with us today due to their early deaths. . . . My legs walk better, even though my right leg has been amputated above the knee, and my ears hear better than those who are no longer with us, even though I am now totally deaf in one ear and have lost 50 percent in the other."

Some of you may think that the term *positive attitudinal healing* sounds pretty fancy or that it is strictly a bunch of bunk, or you may already know a lot about it. I refer you to *The Healing Brain*, edited by Robert Ornstein and Charles Swencionis, which details the scientific studies that have revealed evidence of the various psychological states and life traumas that can adversely affect the immune system. There is much scientific evidence in support of this theory. Eminent psychiatrists, psychologists, and neuroscientists describe investigations into the mind-brain-body relationships that are changing our understanding of the illness process. It is fascinating reading.

I am a believer in a healthy, positive attitude and that we can deal with the most negative aspects of diabetes in a positive manner. Think about it for a minute. If we choose to deal with the negative aspects of diabetes negatively, then we end up with a compound problem, because the negative mind-set adds a new dimension to the powerful deleterious effects. It is indeed true that we must at some point deal with the negative side of diabetes, so why not approach this particular aspect in the most positive manner humanly possible? If you continuously program for a negative result, then most likely you will, sooner or later, achieve a negative result. Conversely, if you program yourself for a positive result, then, even if you do not fully realize your goal, at least you will be mentally prepared for the eventual outcome and will be more mentally and physically adept at handling whatever result may occur.

It is my experience that diabetes responds best to this positive mental attitude. Your diabetes is a very real part of your life, and it will not go away. Is it not easier to live with if you accept only positive attitudes and thoughts to become part of your daily living? There is an abundance of books at your local library or bookstore on all the various aspects of positive thinking. Pick up some of these books and find a plan that is best suited for you. The important thing is to make it work for your life and not be fooled into thinking that super miracles will happen immediately. If you think this way, however, miracles happen every day, so why not program your positive mental resources to produce miracles for you? It seems to me that most of us expect the worst things to happen and program our minds in a negative way rather than a positive one. Remember, miracles happen; it is just that we have become jaded in our regard of what a true miracle really is. Have you ever stopped to think of the absolute miracle a newborn baby represents? How about the fact that even though your pancreas does not work, you are able to inject the modern miracle of genetically engineered human insulin to enable you to remain alive? Yes, there are problems associated in remaining alive with diabetes, but would you really prefer the alternative?

Instead of selling you on developing a healthy positive attitude, I would rather have you see the difference for yourself. The O. Carl Simonton, M.D., Cancer Counseling and Research Center in Fort Worth, Texas (see page 181), is known worldwide for their belief and practice of positive right-brain healing using alpha brain biorhthyms. It is these folks who pioneered the mental imagery of the white knights, the good white blood cells, fighting off and killing the black knights, the bad cancer cells. The power of this visual "mind" energy is awesome, yet it remains an untapped resource by many who are unaware of its positive energy. Many people have been sent to the Simonton Center as a last resort. Many who have opened their minds and tried their best to follow the positive attitudinal healing program have left the clinic in better health. Those who have preprogrammed themselves to die most certainly die.

This is not to say that some of those with the positive mind-set did not also die, but perhaps their quality of life improved, even though it was indeed their time to pass away. I believe that this new area of medicine, wherein the mind is called upon to instruct the brain to send healing chemicals and mechanisms to "cure" the sick organ, tissue, or cellular component, all of which is a mystery to us now, may someday be the new age of enlightened medicine.

Albert Einstein, my hero since I was a child, said that we only use 5–8 percent of our brain. Can you imagine the superior intellect and mental ability you could have if you were able to double or triple the amount of brain you actively use on a daily basis? Now consider for a moment that you were trained to use a method in which you could use more of your brain. Many scientists today think that the way to find this ability is to learn to use the right brain. The right brain is the intuitive side of the brain, whereas the left brain is more prone to accomplish the everyday tasks that must be carried out in the normal functioning of our human bodies. Many experiments have been carried out over the years, using sensitive instruments called electroencephalographs, or EEG machines, that enable a doctor to study the brain frequencies and their role in human functioning. The brain can be likened to a radio transmitter. It operates on specific frequencies and with specific voltages. When we are born, our brains begin functioning at the alpha brain-wave frequency. This is a relatively midrange frequency of about seven to fourteen cycles, or hertz. As we get older, into adolescence and teenage years, and then on into adulthood, our brains begin running more in the beta range of frequencies, about fourteen to twenty-one hertz and above. Researchers have found that the most beneficial brain-wave functioning is in the alpha range. As adults, with the many stresses involved in everyday life, the beta brain-wave functioning seems to work to get us by. However, for real problem solving, the brain-wave frequency of the alpha range has been found to be far superior, as it is in this frequency range that more of the genius qualities are derived. There is much speculation and theorizing that is being done in this area of the mind because there are so many facets of the human brain and mind that defy our understanding.

Let us say that we could enter into an alpha state of brain-wave frequency and instruct our brain to better heal our bodies or better prepare us for an examination in school, or any myriad of other life problems for which we need good solutions. I have carried out experiments on myself using alpha brain-wave frequencies. Achieving alpha brain-wave frequencies is a learned response. At one point in your life you had to learn how to swim before it became a natural experience. Think of the awkwardness learning to ride a bicycle presented the first time you tried. It is much the same in learning how to engage the inner consciousness level of the right brain and the alpha state of brain-wave frequencies. Once you learn the proper technique and practice every day, then you too may derive beneficial results. Open your mind and study the various methods that appear in books today.

Eight million graduates of Silva International from all over the world have learned that this enlightened look at the human body, through better control of the right brain, has an influence on the human body, spirituality, and the betterment of life. If you stop and consider the multifaceted aspect to the better understanding of the mind-brain-body approach to healing of not only the physical self but also the mental and spiritual self, I think you will find a deep solace in this work. Check it out for yourself and see if you will be able to benefit from a deeper consciousness level of understanding.

A French physician, Emile Coue, came to the United States around 1920. He saw many sick people, and for many he gave the same prescription. On his prescription blank he recommended that his patients repeat the following phrase twenty times in the morning and twenty times before bedtime: "Every day in every way, I am getting better, better, and better." The positive attitudinal healing process that this simple prescription set up achieved amazing results. I certainly am not trying to knock modern pharmacology, but why not utilize both modern drug therapy and positive attitudinal healing to enrich whatever therapy is prescribed? I use higher mental power to help me in my daily ups and downs with diabetes. And remember, we are trying our best to live and get the most out of life in dealing positively with the daily illness of insulin-dependent and non-insulin-dependent diabetes mellitus.

I learned the Silva technique from my friend, Hank Belopavlovich, so that I could utilize the right brain and alpha brain-wave frequencies to better deal with my diabetes. At the time he was teaching me the course, my diabetes had taken a turn for the worse, due to personal problems with an intimate relationship. The woman and I had parted company and I was suffering from depression and a further negative outlook on my future. A routine blood chemistry, taken before I began the course with Hank, indicated that my blood glucose average control for a three-month period was poor, as measured by a hemoglobin A_1C test. My cholesterol levels were high and my blood fats were also high. My renal function, as measured by creatinine clearance and glomerular filtration rate, was also poor. What did I have to lose by trying something at this point in my life that my conservative medical training would have never permitted me to do before? I began using the techniques of positive attitudinal healing and right-brain alpha states. Three months later, I had another routine blood chemistry. This time the picture looked better than it had in years. My kidney function was excellent, as was my blood glucose control average. My cholesterol had fallen below two hundred and my blood fats were below one hundred. Every aspect looked so good that my doctor could not believe he was seeing the blood chemistry of a long-term, totally blind, diabetic patient. Was this due to my new application of alpha states and positive healing through using the right brain? Scientifically and objectively, I honestly cannot say for sure. However, the results made me very happy and showed a tremendous positive change over the rather grim results of the previous test, when I was not using these techniques. So, I continue to use these techniques every day. Why not? If you were to come up to me today and ask, "Hey, how are you doing?" I am very likely to reply, "Oh, just fine, better and better. How about yourself?"

Modern medicine is as interested in the mind-brain-body relationship and the immune system as it is concerned with the overall illness process. The effects of stress alone in the United States, with its link to strokes and heart attacks, is staggering. Think about how much better off you could be if you could learn some of the mental steps that would enable you to relax and become more stress-free. Believe me, it could save your life.

I believe you must do everything possible and use all the mental power you can muster to deal with diabetes on a daily basis. Of course, it goes without saying that you must be mindful of quick cures and quack remedies. Do not misunderstand for one second what I am trying to get across to you here. Good common sense and logic are always your best armaments in dealing with anything you feel will not honestly be of benefit to your better health.

13

Exercise Physiology and Diabetes

The importance of exercise to the metabolism and hormonal control of diabetes goes all the way back to 600 B.C., when the Indian physician Seshruta prescribed it as an important adjunct to controlling some types of diabetes. Exercise was well recognized as a therapeutic tool to aid in the control of diabetes during the eighteenth century, but by 1798 the physician John Rollo recommended that his more severe diabetic patients be confined to bed rest, at least until there was considerable improvement. Slightly more than one hundred years ago the important role of exercise in the treatment of diabetes was emphasized again. After the discovery of insulin in 1922, exercise joined insulin and diet as one of the three important factors used to control diabetes.

Up until the last twenty years, there was little scientific evidence to support the validity of exercise for the diabetic patient. Research has since shown that exercise is vitally important in the control of diabetes.

Sports and exercise played an important role in preserving my life as a young teenager. My diabetes was undiagnosed and uncontrolled. During this two-year period when my diabetes was becoming more and more blatant, I began karate lessons; this demanding physical training program helped me survive during prolonged, extremely high blood glucose levels. Finally, my mother insisted on a blood chemistry test (blood chemistries were not routine thirty years ago). I was diagnosed and was given my first life-saving insulin injection.

Because I feel that the martial arts helped save my life, I continue training today. I achieved a black belt while in Hawaii and have studied Japanese shoto kan, Korean tae kwon do, and the special style of Korean to kong moo so. The martial arts teach discipline, humility, respect, and powerful techniques of self-defense. If you are looking for a sport that you can stay with for the rest of your life, then consider the martial arts. A high-level Oriental master will teach you the philosophy of martial arts, not just how to break a board or brick with your hand.

When I became totally blind due to complications of diabetic retinopathy, my beloved surfing and other sports programs came to an abrupt end. While in rehabilitation, I engaged in a light exercise program that included walking on a treadmill, using a rowing machine and several other machines, and doing exercises to give myself a cardiovascular workout. With my excellent mobility instructor, Suzie Nagle, still my dear friend today, I was taught to use a white cane; daily walks of one mile or more helped to provide additional exercise.

As I became more accustomed to blindness, I began my martial arts training again, this time practicing to kong moo so, a difficult style encompassing twenty-six different martial arts styles, including akido, jujitsu, escrima, judo, tae kwon do, and use of all the martial arts weapons from nunchakus to samurai swords. This was a wonderful source of training for me because my Oriental grand master, who developed this style and taught it to the Korean special forces, had himself been trained by a blind master.

I decided I needed an exercise machine that I could work out on at home without worrying about inclement weather, getting to the martial arts training facility, and so on. After carefully studying exercise machines for home use, four years ago I ordered a Nordic-Track cross-country skiing machine.

I thought I was in pretty good shape until I did my first fifteen minutes on the NordicTrack. It does take some getting used to, but once I found my balance points, I began strengthening muscles. I can work out for an hour on this machine today. My NordicTrack was one of the best single investments I have made in terms of improving my cardiovascular system and stamina, reducing my weight, and trimming off unwanted inches, while adding bulk to my shoulders and girth to my chest.

Cross-country skiing was developed by northern Europeans and Scandinavians in order to get from point to point in deep snow.

They strapped wooden skis to their boots, allowing for more accessible transportation and hunting during the winter months. As modern industrialization began taking place, cross-country skiing made the transition from utility to sport.

Cross-country skiing is an excellent aerobic exercise to improve or maintain cardiovascular fitness because it requires both arm and leg work, thus realizing a high level of energy expenditure. It is one of the most demanding of the endurance sports because it uses muscles in the shoulders, back, chest, legs, abdomen, and buttocks. Cross-country skiing athletes easily burn in excess of one thousand calories per hour, and Dr. Kenneth Cooper, founder of the aerobics movement, rates cross-country skiing as the top cardiorespiratory activity in terms of its overall exercise value. It has been scientifically determined by exercise physiologists that this type of exercise provides tremendous benefit for the cardiovascular system because it provides the muscles with a continuous stream of oxygen and nutrients so that high energy output can be maintained for a considerable period of time.

During the very cold Minnesota winter of 1975, a mechanical device was designed to simulate cross-country skiing while indoors, and so the NordicTrack was born. Some excellent research data has been accumulated at the University of Wisconsin–La Crosse, the University of Minnesota, and the University of Massachusetts to support use of the NordicTrack cross-country skiing machine. These data are available from the NordicTrack Company (see Other Resources, page 180, should you want to do additional study). I have been impressed with the tremendous aerobic benefit the NordicTrack provides over the stationary bicycle and the treadmill. Check into this area yourself and, as always, consult with your doctor before engaging into any strenuous exercise program. Also, carefully monitor your blood glucose levels.

I have found that good cardiovascular fitness is not achieved by some sort of magical, painless technique. It requires some effort and dedication, but it is not necessary to drive oneself to exhaustion every workout to achieve good results. In other words, stimulation is necessary, but excess is not necessarily better.

Thanks to my NordicTrack machine, I have been able to maintain a regular training schedule even when it is raining or snowing or the temperatures are soaring in the high nineties. But exercise must be continued on a regular basis. A significant reduction in cardiovascular fitness occurs after as little as two weeks of inactivity; a loss of up to 50 percent of initial improvement in aerobic capacity has been shown after four to twelve weeks of inactivity.

I have found that my blood glucose does tend to be higher in the mornings after one hour of vigorous exercise on the NordicTrack exercise machine. I can expect an increase of 50–100 mg/dl on my morning blood glucose test after exercise. At first I was puzzled when my tests were higher than expected each morning after exercise, until I reviewed the exercise physiology literature concerning experimental data for diabetic animals.

If my morning fasting blood glucose reading is, for example, 135 mg/dl without exercise, after one hour of vigorous exercise my glucose reading may be 225 mg/dl. This should be kept in mind if you exercise in the morning before taking your insulin or oral antidiabetic medication. Conversely, if you take your insulin after measuring your fasting blood glucose level in the morning, then engage in your vigorous exercise routine, you must be especially careful to avoid going into a hypoglycemic reaction. This is true whether you have eaten or not, but is very dangerous if you have chosen to take your insulin or oral meds, do not eat, and then exercise. Unless your morning blood glucose level is very high, taking your insulin without eating and then engaging in a vigorous exercise program could be very dangerous. I make it a practice never to do this. It has been proven that insulin, when injected subcutaneously, is absorbed more rapidly into the circulation when muscles underlying the injection site are contracted, as in vigorous exercise.

In terms of biochemistry and physiology, there are some complex phenomena involved. These are advanced biochemical and physiological theories and models involved with the uptake of insulin and glucose into muscles. Studies using insulin-dependent dogs have proved that after vigorous exercise, blood glucose levels rise sharply twenty-eight hours after the last insulin dose. It was reported that this observation was due to an increase in glucose production rates, while glucose utilization remained constant. This means that during vigorous exercise, the glucose utilized by muscles continues at a steady pace of uptake. Further experiments showed that vigorous exercise actually failed to adequately stimulate the peripheral utilization of insulin.

In terms of conditioning, exercise stresses the body and the body adapts to the stress by getting stronger and leaner and by acquiring the physical and emotional underpinnings of greater endurance. A state of mild fatigue is achieved when the individual overloads his system by stressing more than usual. A period of recovery takes place during which the body responds to the stimulation by adapting up to a level of function that is greater than the beginning level. Exercise continued before too much regression takes place allows the cycle to repeat, thus achieving and maintaining good cardiovascular fitness.

Experts agree that to achieve this kind of overload on the cardiovascular system, a heart rate target zone of 60–85 percent of maximum heart rate is effective in eliciting an aerobic training effect. To determine a rough estimate of maximum heart rate, subtract your age in years from 220. For example, a forty-year-old man would have a maximum heart rate of 180 beats per minute.

An aerobically fit person exhibits a reduced heart rate both at rest and at any given submaximal (below maximum) exercise intensity. The quantity of blood pumped with each heartbeat is increased, the size of the heart increases, and the heart becomes a more efficient muscle overall. For diabetics the most important aspect is the fact that as one exercises, capillary density increases (up to 40 percent), enabling more oxygen, hormones, and nutrients to be delivered to the muscles. Aerobic training increases the ability of the muscles to utilize oxygen and to use glycogen (stored glucose, the immediate energy source of muscles).

Nearly fifty-eight million Americans have high blood pressure, many of these with Type I or Type II diabetes. Because high blood pressure is the single most important risk factor for stroke, with even mild elevations doubling the risk, and because diabetes is a risk factor for high blood pressure, heart attack, and stroke, it is extremely important that we not only monitor our blood pressure, but do everything possible to keep it under control.

Blood pressure is the force exerted by the blood against the arterial walls. When you or your doctor takes your blood pressure reading, for example 120/80 mm Hg, the top number is the systolic pressure, the pressure exerted against the artery walls, and the bottom number is the diastolic pressure, which is the lowest pressure remaining in the arteries between heartbeats when the heart is at rest. Blood pressure is considered high when the systolic blood pressure is over 140 and the diastolic blood pressure is over 90. Consult with your doctor concerning your level of blood pressure control, as this area is vitally important to the life of the diabetic. Regular aerobic exercise may reduce the resting blood pressure, especially for those whose blood pressure is elevated.

Here are some simple exercises you can do with little strain and pain.

1. Upside-Down Butterfly

Upon rising in the morning, lie down flat on your back on the floor, with your arms at your side. Raise your legs about twelve inches in the air, with feet together. Keeping your legs in the air, raise and lower your arms rapidly in counts of five. With a count of five, while raising and lowering your arms rapidly, breathe in for the full count. Repeat with the next count of five while exhaling. Breathe in through the nose; exhale through the mouth. Work your way to a count of one hundred.

2. Leaf Curl

While lying flat on your back, stretch out fully and place your outstretched arms above your head. Begin lifting your head and back while tightening your stomach muscles. Continue pulling yourself forward, with your legs together and flat on the floor, until you stretch out and try to touch your toes. Slowly uncurl yourself, with stomach muscles tight, as you continue back to the starting position. Do these slowly and carefully so as not to pull a hamstring. Do at least ten repetitions.

3. Ups and Downs

While drying your hair or shaving, go up and down on your toes for a count of one hundred. Do these slowly to get maximum benefit for the toes, feet, and calf muscles.

4. Rock Stomach
While drying your hair or shaving, take in a deep breath of air through the nose. Hold it in and tighten the stomach muscles for a count of twenty. Do as many repetitions as time will allow.

5. Steering Wheel Crush
We have gotten through the morning while you are getting ready to go to work. Now you are in your car with nothing to do but listen to the stereo. Why not some dynamic muscle tension? Grab the steering wheel tightly and push inward with both hands. Tighten the stomach muscles and practice adding force from the inner arms to the shoulders.

6. Coffee Break Escape
While the rest of your office bunch heads to the coffeepot at break time, head down the hallway and outside for a brisk walk around the building. On your way back into your office, get that cup of coffee and drink it at your desk.

7. Desk Lift
While at your desk, place both hands under the front of your desk. Lift with both hands as if to raise the desk toward the ceiling. Tighten your stomach muscles as you do so.

8. Leg Stretch
Every hour or so during a busy day at your desk, stretch your legs tightly for a count of twenty. Release and relax completely. Try to make this a habit so as to increase the circulation of the legs. By the way, make sure your office chair does not have a ridge at the edge where your legs can become restricted, causing circulation problems for the diabetic. If this is so, ask for another chair.

8. Don't Forget to Breathe
Whenever you can think of it, try to take in a deep breath through the nose and hold it for as long as you can. Exhale thoroughly through the mouth. Repeat a few times and you will notice a renewed feeling just through the oxygenation process. Many times we are so stressed out at work, we simply forget to breathe.

9. Crow's Neck Stretch
Turn your head as far to the left as you can. After you have reached this point, stretch it farther to the left. Do the same for the right. Repeat this several times to loosen the neck muscles and relieve neck strain.

10. Twist and Shout
While standing, place arms in front with hands clasped together. Twist the upper torso from left to right while keeping the legs together and straight ahead. The shout is optional, but it sure does relieve a lot of built-up stress!

This is certainly not an exhaustive list of exercises, but it will give you an idea of some of the things you can do to utilize any spare moment available. Perhaps you are already involved in a physical fitness program that you are comfortable with and works well for you. The important thing to remember here is that exercise is vital in the management of your diabetes. If you are only able to do a few of the exercises listed above on a daily basis, then you are still better off than the diabetic who does absolutely nothing.

My exercise program makes me feel so good that it is a joyful beginning to every day. This is crucial for me emotionally and psychologically, as I believe that daily exercise is life-extending for the diabetic.

14

Acupuncture and Diabetes

Acupuncture became a topic of great interest and debate in the United States in the early 1970s. A number of books appeared on the market and interest in this ancient Oriental medical practice became intense. I eagerly read all the available books on the subject and studied the meridians that had been mapped out by the Chinese over seven thousand years ago.

Unfortunately for me, I did not have any kind of acupuncture treatment until two and a half years ago, when I was introduced to a school of Chinese medicine. Due to acupuncture's advantageous effect on the microcirculation, I might have derived a great benefit at the time of my diabetic retinopathy through the application of Chinese acupuncture and herbal medicine to give me relief from the tremendous physical pain I was suffering, pain that Western medications could not alleviate. If I had begun acupuncture treatments before I began losing my eyesight, I believe that my case of diabetes would be in even better shape today.

Oriental medicine and Western medicine each has its own distinct advantages. For example, Western medicine has in its arsenal an abundance of medications, which, if given antisymptomatically, are helpless in preventing migraine headaches and reducing the symptoms unless one continues to take the medication. But I have witnessed intractable migraine headaches virtually disappear with a series of acupuncture treatments. An immovable shoulder joint accompanied by severe pain is usually not affected by traditional Western medicine treatment other than relief of pain through the use of steroid hormones on a continuing basis. The use of these steroid hormones may create side effects that include moon face, osteoporosis, ulcerative conditions of the stomach and gastric mucosa, cataracts, glaucoma, and immune-system failure. Again, I have seen patients come for just one acupuncture treatment and achieve almost miraculous results with their shoulder or other affected joint. The microvasculature of the brain is vastly improved through enhanced circulation, which in turn improves symptoms of irritability, short-term memory loss, and insomnia in the elderly.

What is so important for the diabetic to learn about acupuncture is the improvement to the microcirculation deep within the microvasculature of the body. As we have learned in the chapters on the eye, kidney, nervous system, and heart, it is the microvessels that fall prone to the insidious nature of diabetes, for reasons we still do not fully understand. Importantly, the improvements acupuncture provides to the microcirculation mean a lessened tendency toward high blood pressure in those individuals with hypertension. In addition, acupuncture induces a series of blood chemistry changes, such as a decrease in serum triglyceride and phospholipid levels, a mild decrease in serum cholesterol level, an increase in ACTH and cortisol, and a normalization of abnormal levels and quality of red blood cells and white blood cells, among many other blood chemistry changes.

Acupuncture is to a large degree ineffectual in the treatment of infectious diseases. Because diabetics, especially when not well controlled, can be prone to infections, Western medicine is superior in this respect when appropriate antibiotics are utilized. Certainly, then, if the Western medical doctor were also trained to use acupuncture, the best of both worlds could then be used to offer the best treatment to the diabetic, or any patient.

I have been taking weekly acupuncture treatments for over two years now. My right eye, with ten years of blindness, had begun to develop what is known as microophthalmia due to the blindness itself and atrophy. This is a condition common to blind diabetics. In simple terms, it means that the eyeball is becoming smaller and smaller. I knew this condition was occurring; however, my family was reluctant to inform me because of the possible stress it could cause. In addition to microophthalmia, the eye, instead of looking healthy, was looking lifeless. I decided to try acupuncture for treatment to improve the condition of my right eye.

The Chinese doctors who knew of diabetes knew there was

little hope of returning vision, short of a miracle. However, they attempted to reconnect vital forces that became blocked during my initial onset of diabetic retinopathy. Every week the clinical instructor, a master acupuncturist, Dr. Jeff Tsing, would work painstakingly on my right eye. He inserted needles deep into the orbit socket under, above, and to each side of the eye, never placing a needle close to the eye itself. After several months of treatments, my family began to notice an incredible change in my right eye. It had gained volume, making it appear more normal in size in relation to my left eye. The right eye appeared to take on new life and began to look and feel more normal than it had in years.

Knowing this now as a medical fact, with my clinic records as proof, I began thinking about the possibilities of improving the microcirculation of the eyes during the initial onset of diabetic retinopathy. Why couldn't we have some experimental protocols developed to use the best of our Western medical techniques and acupuncture to treat this insidious disease? Would it be possible to develop a rational therapy of the use of acupuncture, lasers, and the new generation of antiretinopathy drugs to stop its devastation?

After this incredible improvement to my right eye, I decided to ask my acupuncturist to engage upon a program of treatments to improve my kidney function and to help me in preventing diabetic nephropathy and end-stage renal disease. I am happy to report normal kidney function at this time, and I will continue to use acupuncture treatments, perhaps for the rest of my life, so that the microvasculature in all parts of my body is eventually improved.

When the acupuncturist inserts a needle, there is little or no pain felt. Depending upon your own particular treatment regimen, the acupuncturist will then stimulate the insertion point by rapid up-and-down movements or by rotating the needle until the correct placement is found. An electrifying jolt down or up the nerve pathway assures the acupuncturist that he or she has attained the correct placement. I have feelings of light euphoria after an acupuncture treatment and the sessions usually last thirty to forty-five minutes, allowing for restful meditation while the treatment produces its rather mystical effect.

The nerve conductance in my feet and legs has vastly improved. I can feel nerve impulses rush like a bolt of electricity to the tips of my toes and soles of my feet when needle stimulation is applied to my legs or the tops of my feet. While training with a martial arts cane, I was rapidly swinging the cane in figure-eight patterns; while slowing down the cane, it lightly touched the inside of my knee joint. Later that night I could not walk due to the intractable pain. Fortunately, my acupuncture treatment was set for the next week, and I mentioned to Dr. Tsing the amount of pain I was suffering in my knee. He placed two needles in very specific areas of the knee and proceeded to treat me for the diabetic condition as he normally does. After approximately forty minutes on the table, I found that there was no pain remaining in my knee. I really could not believe it, so I did a mental inventory while I walked to the front of the clinic in order to see if I had just psyched out the pain. The pain was actually gone, and I have not suffered any pain of the knee joint since the mishap occurred.

In addition to its other benefits, there is an economic consideration for the use of acupuncture. In the case of the immovable shoulder joint and the migraine headache, the patient may have to see a physician once or twice a week, and this may continue for a lifetime. The cost involved for this type of treatment is considerable, and if the patient cannot work, the economic burden becomes even greater. However, acupuncture can eliminate most of these problems with just a few treatments or a series of treatments over several months; the economic burden is much less.

In Japan, China, and Korea, the use of acupuncture and other types of Oriental medicine is widespread. The lowering of total national medical expense is generally attributable to acupuncture, thus making it possible for every citizen of China and Japan to have national health insurance and free medical care for the elderly over the age of sixty-five.

Acupuncture is part of the ancient Far Eastern Oriental medicine. Oriental medicine is based on the following unique methods of diagnosis:

The physician first examines the patient by the following four methods of examination:

Visual examination with special emphasis on inspection of various parts of the body believed to represent the condition of specific internal organs. These areas include the face, tongue, around the nose, and eyes.

Examination by listening. This includes not only sounds coming from the body, but also smelling of body odors, such as breath, or of excretion.

Examination by questioning. A unique aspect of this line of questioning is that the patient is always asked about any changes in preference to the taste of food.

Examination by palpation. This begins with an overall examination of pulses of three representative parts of the body, which are the face, the hands, and the feet. Some practitioners also examine the carotid arteries, followed by other methods of palpation of other areas of the body.

The Oriental practitioner then classifies the symptoms of the patient into four pairs of opposing syndromes: Yin and Yang; deep and superficial; empty and full; cold and hot.

Once all of the patient's symptoms have been classified into the four categories of these eight choices of categories of syndromes, the appropriate treatment is chosen between acupuncture with supplemental moxibustion, or moxibustion as the main treatment with acupuncture used only supplementally. Moxibustion is the addition of an herb, moxa, to a special needle; the herb is ignited, which produces heat transfer down the needle. This treatment is termed "treatment based on the classification of syndromes" and forms the basis of the Oriental medical practice.

Acupuncture is only one part of Far Eastern Oriental medicine, which includes herbology and the use of nonherb medicines, herbal elixirs, acupuncture, moxibustion, cupping, certain types of massage, breath regulation, exercises based on five different animals (tiger, deer, bear, monkey, bird), harmonious sexual life and strong sexual potency, prevention of aging and achieving long life.

The term *acupuncture* actually comes from the Greek, acus, meaning needle, and punctura, meaning puncture. Acupuncture has been used for many centuries in Oriental countries, particularly Japan, China, and Korea. The oldest description of acupuncture comes from the book *Nei Ching*, most probably written in the second or third century B.C. in China.

Chi Energy

The concept of chi, pronounced "key," energy forms the basis of Oriental medicine. Chi is the important vital energy flowing in a certain predetermined direction from one meridian to another meridian, circulating through the entire body of humans or animals. Chi can be spelled Qi, ch'i (the proper Chinese spelling), or ki (Japanese). When the flow of chi is in excess, is lacking, or is unbalanced, this is considered to be an abnormal state of the body, requiring adjustments in relation to other symptoms or syndromes as determined by the practitioner. Any abnormality of the vital energy flow of chi is considered to produce diseases. Acupuncture points are utilized to correct the vital energy flow of chi.

In ancient China, around the first or second century B.C., medical practitioners knew of twelve internal organs, and it was believed that these organs had specific connections to distal parts of the body, such as the extremities or the head. This imaginary line of connection between each internal organ and the corresponding outer part of the body was called ching, meaning vein or artery. Ching was earlier translated by the French to mean meridian. Meridian is now known all over the world as one of the important concepts within Oriental medicine and acupuncture.

There are twelve principle meridians that correspond to the six yin internal organs and the six yang internal organs. Eight additional meridians were described in the ancient text *Nei Ching*, and these meridians do not have any direct connection to any one of the twelve internal organs. These additional meridians are also known as odd meridians, irregular vessels, and curious meridians. The study of the meridians, as you may suspect, becomes more intriguing and difficult as you delve into Oriental philosophy. The ancient Chinese were so meticulous in the mapping of the meridians that, as of a few years ago, our high-technology medicine, using infrared spectroscopy, has determined them to be correct.

A series of acupuncture points, that is, where the needles are actually inserted, is found on each meridian of each one of the twelve internal organs of the classical Chinese concept. Current Oriental medical practice does not limit acupuncture points to the meridians; the practitioner determines additional points by palpation and other means of physical examination.

The ancient acupuncturists, practicing a more primitive form of acupuncture, used needles made of flint, stone, sharpened bamboo, bronze, or gold. The oldest acupuncture needles, found in the ancient graveyard of the historically significant acupuncture specialists, were made of gold and had a shaft diameter of more than two millimeters. Due to the thickness of the bore of the needles used at that time, there was probably a great deal of pain involved.

Today's acupuncture needles come in a variety of sizes, depending on the amount of body fat, the depth of insertion, and other applications. Acupuncture needles are used only once, each needle contained in a separate sterile package. The entire procedure is painless and the feelings after the treatment are of slight euphoria.

For me, the study of acupuncture and Oriental medicine is as fascinating and boundless as the study of our Western medicine. The health benefits I have attained through the use of acupuncture treatments are inestimable in all areas of my health, including improved sexual libido and performance. Students of acupuncture have their patients' total health as the prime objective at all times.

If you have a school of Chinese medicine or have access to a practitioner of Oriental medicine or acupuncture, consider trying the treatment for improvement of your diabetes. As always, discuss with your own doctor any medical changes you plan to initiate. Your doctor may want to study any benefits derived from acupuncture by reviewing blood chemistry results before you begin treatments and, for instance, after a two- or three-month series of treatments. Whatever choice you make, I hope you have as much success as I have had with this ancient Oriental practice.

15

The Diabetic Diet

One of the first items a newly diagnosed diabetic must deal with is the diabetic diet, its theory, mechanics, and manipulations. The diabetic exchange list is introduced, as well as how important this list is to the regime. The Diabetic Exchange List, developed jointly by the American Diabetes Association and the American Dietetic Association in the early 1960s and revised in 1986, forms the backbone of the diabetic diet. Using the exchange list, you can substitute one food for another based on the breakdown of the substituted food in terms of carbohydrates, fats, protein, and sugar. From this list your individual diet can be tailored to meet your activity level, the amount of insulin or oral antidiabetic medication you take, your age group, your own specific caloric requirements, and your own particular lifestyle. As you become more familiar with the exchange list and the meal plan, you will develop a better understanding of the manipulations that are possible. This understanding will help you manage your new diet, but it will require time, study, patience, and a good positive attitude.

As I look back some thirty-two years, I can recall my feelings when I first learned about my new diabetic diet. One of the grinding dilemmas that confronted my family and me when I was first diagnosed was the emotional overload of being told I would have to be on a very special, restricted diet for the rest of my life and that this diet would be an integral part of the therapy designed to prolong my life. I became very depressed when told that this diet would restrict me from any and all the items that make a meal appetizing and appealing.

The diabetic manuals of thirty years ago listed columns of restricted food. I would play games with this and recite the long list of restricted items. My family would look at me and just wonder what it was, exactly, that I *could* eat. Of course, everything with sugar was either restricted entirely or limited to minute quantities. After some time, my mother figured that I could eat green beans, onions, lettuce, cucumbers, and other vegetables containing few calories, in unlimited quantities. Even while I was in the hospital getting regulated to my insulin requirements, one of the staples at lunch and dinner was an onion salad consisting of sliced onions and vinegar, a combination that is just not very tasty. No oil or salad dressing was added to this little salad, and even today I will break out in a cold sweat when I think of a vinegar-only salad dressing. In fact, the tendency to get violent enters my mind.

The hospital food-service staff tried their best to serve me decent meals during my stay, but the diabetic diet at that time was very limited and certainly not creative. For breakfast, there were powdered eggs cooked without even a hint of butter, limp white bread toast with a drop of margarine, skim milk that was blue in color and had the consistency of water, and, if I was lucky, a strip or two of bacon that had been sacrificed to the fire gods. Thirty years ago, dieticians and nutritionists knew that foods high in fat and sugar were definitely not good for the diabetic.

Now take a look at what nutritionists recommend for the general health of the average nondiabetic American today. It looks suspiciously like the new diabetic diet. Over the years, I have often wondered what would have happened if, over twenty-five years ago, everyone was placed on a diabetic diet. Would we see such an overabundance of clogged arteries, coronary artery disease, arteriosclerosis, and stroke? Would the general population be trimmer, less lethargic, and less overweight? I regard the improved diabetic diet as a very health-conscious diet, and it is interesting that the American Heart Association and the American Cancer Society recommend diets closely resembling today's diabetic diet.

In any diabetic management program, diet plays a crucial role. If you are non-insulin-dependent and carefully manage your diet, your diabetes may become less severe and the possibility exists that your diabetes may disappear altogether. This will require tremendous determination and discipline on your part. Typically, a non-insulin-dependent diabetic will begin a diet with a valiant effort at first; then the tendency to pick up the old habits of eating everything and in the wrong quantities becomes greater and greater. This of course includes eating more things such as pies, cakes, and sweets, which means that additional weight is gained, so oral medication must be increased due to higher blood sugar values, thus creating a vicious cycle.

For those of us who are insulin-dependent, with strict dietary management and exercise and careful regulation of our blood sugar and insulin intake, we too can benefit, in terms of lowering our insulin requirements and maintaining less body fat, and thus, hopefully, preventing or delaying the onset of long-term complications.

Here are the nutrition therapy recommendations published by the American Diabetes Association in 1997. Because the nutritional requirements of the diabetic are complex and new information is forthcoming all the time, I agree with the American Diabetes Association when they recommend that a registered dietician, knowledgeable in the nutritional requirements of the diabetic, be part of your health care team. Since the last publication of a position statement by the American Diabetes Association in 1991, several items have been reconsidered and make up the main emphasis of this new statement for 1997.

Over the last several years, it had been thought that increasing carbohydrate intake was okay for the diabetic and that diabetics as well as marathon runners and those engaging in extreme sports could benefit from a diet rich in complex carbohydrates including large amounts of pasta, beans, potatoes, and rice. However, the newest findings indicate that this intake leads to higher blood glucose values and weight gain, so it is now recommended that the diabetic carefully monitor the amount of simple and complex carbohydrates consumed.

Goals of Nutrition Therapy for the Diabetic

Maintenance of good blood glucose control is of prime importance and can be achieved by balancing food intake with insulin, oral antidiabetic medications, and exercise and activity levels.

We want to work toward achievement of optimal serum lipid levels. These levels are monitored by your doctor when he or she draws a blood sample and sends it to the lab (see Chapter 5 on clinical blood tests).

The adult should maintain adequate weight or achieve a weight appropriate and reasonable to the individual through proper caloric intake. Reasonable weight is defined as the weight an individual and his health care provider acknowledge as achievable and maintainable, not necessarily the traditionally defined desirable or ideal body weight.

Individuals with diabetes and their family members should study the USDA food pyramid and follow its basic guidelines.

Nutrition Therapy and Type I Diabetes—A meal plan based on the individual's usual food intake should be determined. This normal eating pattern can then be used as a guide for integrating insulin therapy into the individual's usual eating and exercise patterns. Meals should occur at consistent times synchronized with the time-action of the insulin preparation used. Individuals need to monitor blood glucose levels and adjust insulin doses for the amount of food they usually eat. Intensified insulin therapy, such as multiple daily injections or use of an insulin pump, allows flexibility in meal plan timing and content. By using intensified therapy, the individual can integrate insulin regimens with his lifestyle and adjust them for changes from usual eating and exercise habits.

Nutrition Therapy and Type II Diabetes—Of utmost importance to the individual with Type II diabetes is achieving glucose, lipid, and blood pressure goals. Weight loss and low-calorie diets can improve short-term blood glucose levels and have the potential to improve long-term metabolic control. Traditional dietary strategies and even very-low-calorie diets have usually not been successful in achieving long-term weight loss. A greater emphasis should be placed on achieving normalized glucose and lipid levels.

Protein—At the present time, there is insufficient evidence to support protein intakes either higher or lower than the average for the general population, that is, 10–20 percent of the daily caloric intake from protein from both animal and vegetable sources.

However, with the onset of overt nephropathy, a lower protein intake is necessary; 10 percent of daily calories is sufficiently restrictive for individuals with evidence of nephropathy.

Total Fat—If dietary protein contributes 10–20 percent of the total caloric content of the diet, then 80–90 percent of calories remain to be distributed between dietary fat and carbohydrates. Less than 10 percent of these calories should be from saturated fats and up to 10 percent calories from polyunsaturated fats, leaving 60–70 percent of the total calories derived from monounsaturated fats and carbohydrates.

The recommended percentage of calories from fat is dependent on desired glucose, lipid, and weight outcomes. Individuals with normal lipid levels and reasonable weight can follow the USDA Dietary Guidelines for Americans recommendations: less than 30 percent of the calories should be from total fat. Children and adolescents should follow the USDA Dietary Guidelines to encourage normal growth and development.

Saturated Fat and Cholesterol—A reduction in saturated fat and cholesterol consumption is necessary to reduce the risk of cardiovascular disease (CVD). Diabetes is a strong independent risk factor for CVD, over and above the adverse effects of an elevated serum cholesterol. Therefore, less than 10 percent of the daily calories should be from saturated fats, and dietary cholesterol should be limited to 300 mg or less daily.

Carbohydrates and Sweeteners—The percentage of calories from carbohydrates will also vary based on the patient's eating habits and his glucose and lipid goals. For most of this century, the most widely held theory about the dietary treatment of diabetes has been that simple sugars should be avoided and replaced with complex carbohydrates. The reasoning is that sugars are more rapidly digested and absorbed than starches, and they thereby aggravate hyperglycemia to a greater degree. There is, however, very little scientific evidence that supports this assertion. Fruits and milk have been shown to create a lower glycemic response than most starches, and sucrose produces a glycemic response similar to that of the starches in bread, rice, and potatoes. Although various starches do have different glycemic responses, from a clinical perspective the patient's first priority should be the total amount of carbohydrates consumed rather than their source.

Sucrose

Sucrose and sucrose-containing foods must be substituted for other carbohydrates, not simply added to the meal plan. In making such substitutions, you should consider the nutrient content of concentrated sweets and sucrose-containing foods, as well as the presence of other nutrients frequently ingested with sucrose, such as fat.

Fructose

Dietary fructose produces a smaller rise in plasma glucose than the same caloric amounts of sucrose and most starchy carbohydrates. In that regard, fructose may offer an advantage as a sweetening agent in the diabetic diet. However, because of potential adverse effects of large amounts of fructose (i.e., double the usual intake [20 percent of calories] on serum cholesterol and LDL cholesterol), it may not be ideal for all diabetics. People with dyslipidemia should avoid consuming large amounts of fructose, but there is no reason to recommend that people avoid fruits and vegetables, in which fructose occurs naturally, or other fructose-sweetened foods in moderate amounts.

Other nutritive sweeteners

Nutritive sweeteners other than sucrose and fructose include corn sweeteners (such as corn syrup), fruit juice or fruit juice concentrate, honey, molasses, dextrose, and maltose. There is no evidence that these sweeteners have any significant advantage or disadvantage over sucrose in terms of caloric content or glycemic response.

Nonnutritive sweeteners

Saccharin, aspartame, and acesulfame K are approved for use by the FDA in the United States. The FDA also determines an acceptable daily intake for approved food additives, including nonnutritive sweeteners. Nonnutritive sweeteners approved by the FDA are safe for all people with diabetes to consume.

For a complete discussion of sweeteners, both nutritive and nonnutritive, see the chapter "Sweets and Sweeteners" in my *Diabetic's Innovative Cookbook*.

Fiber—Dietary fiber may be beneficial in treating or preventing several gastrointestinal disorders, including colon cancer, and large amounts of soluble fiber have a beneficial effect on serum lipids. There is no reason to believe that people with diabetes would be more or less amenable to these effects than those without diabetes. Therefore, recommended fiber intakes for diabetics are the same as for the general population—that is, daily consumption of a diet containing 20 to 35 g of dietary fiber from a wide variety of food sources.

Sodium—People differ greatly in their sensitivity to sodium and in its effect on their blood pressure. Because it is impractical to assess individual sodium sensitivity, recommended intakes for people with diabetes are the same as for the general population. Some health authorities recommend no more than 3,000 mg per day of sodium, while other authorities recommend no more than 2,400 mg per day.

Alcohol—The same precautions regarding the use of alcohol that apply to the general public also apply to people with diabetes. The Dietary Guidelines for Americans recommends no more than two drinks per day for men.

Micronutrients—Although the American Diabetes Association does not specifically recommend vitamins and supplements for the diabetic whose diet is adequate, I take vitamins on a daily basis in order to help my system fight against the ravages of this disease. (See Chapter 16, page 124 on vitamins.)

Summary—Today there is no one diabetic diet. The recommended diet can be defined only as a dietary prescription based on nutrition assessment and treatment goals. Medical nutrition therapy for people with diabetes should be individualized, with consideration given to usual eating habits and other lifestyle factors.

• • •

The demands of the diabetic diet can seem daunting at first, but there are ways to enjoy a diet that is varied and balanced. I am a strong advocate of vegetables and salads. The tastiest salads take advantage of seasonal vegetables, so learning to buy, clean, and prepare fresh vegetables at the peak of ripeness is important. One of my favorite salads, which I lived on during my college days in Hawaii and later in medical school, is my Hawaiian Surfer's Salad. I use one tomato, one-half avocado, one peeled cucumber, one carrot, red-tip lettuce, three or four chunks of cheddar cheese, three or four black olives, and two or three slices of onion, all thinly sliced or finely chopped. After placing everything in a large salad bowl, I add two ounces of canned red salmon, drained. I then add lemon juice, Kraft Lite Italian salad dressing, and a small amount of Kraft Catalina French salad dressing for extra taste. You can substitute tuna for salmon, or fresh grilled salmon for canned salmon. I like to eat some type of good crisp wheat crackers or toasted seven-grain whole wheat bread along with it. This salad is a complete meal.

Here are a few other salad suggestions:

Raw cauliflower cut into florets or sliced with Italian dressing or with vinegar and oil adds few calories except for the dressing. You can do the same preparation with raw broccoli, cabbage, cucumbers, radishes, and onions. Chef's salad is another favorite choice of mine, whether I make it myself or order it at a restaurant. When I make my own chef's salad at home, I add my favorite vegetables and some deli turkey meat and low-fat cheese. Or you can add ham, chicken, or tuna salad.

Many supermarket vegetable departments have fresh spinach available. You can make a great salad using spinach leaves alone or in combination with other vegetables. (Be sure to wash the spinach by soaking the leaves in a bowl of cold water.) Also, many stores carry prepackaged cabbage that has been thinly sliced for making cole slaw or a cabbage salad, a perfect choice when you are in a hurry.

Plan your fresh vegetable purchases to last approximately one week in the refrigerator. Wash leaf lettuce immediately and then replace it in the plastic bag it was purchased in to keep it fresh and crisp.

Remember that carrots and beets are high in sugar and must be accounted for on your diet in order to watch calories. Olives are a fat and, yes, are limited on your diet, too. Try to increase your intake of leafy vegetables and salads on a daily basis.

One note of caution: watch carefully the amount of salad dressing you add. In years past, I consumed a tremendous amount of calories by adding huge quantities of rich salad dressings such as blue cheese dressing and Italian dressing made with oil. The beneficial effects of the salad can be diminished when too much salad dressing is added. Substitute lemon juice for a portion of the salad dressing you would normally use. A salad dressing is supposed to dress the salad, not drown it. I was having lunch at a local restaurant some years ago with a good friend of mine, a psychiatrist who worked at the medical school. I eagerly piled my plate high with everything available at the salad bar and I heaped, just as eagerly, a large amount of blue cheese dressing onto my salad. My friend eyed my plate with amazement and a little disdain. He said, "Man, I guess you are having all your fat exchanges for the week in one salad, huh?" I gave him a rather sharp look, as if to tell him, "Hey, what are you talking about? There is no fat in this salad. Besides, what does a shrink know about fat exchanges anyway?" But he was entirely right. I had become accustomed to eating large quantities of fattening salad dressing, telling myself subconsciously that it was okay since I was eating all those salad greens. It took an objective observer to wake me up. Salad dressing is an important aspect of eating a salad due to the stimulatory effect it has on the production of stomach enzymes, thus leading to better digestion, but it can be highly caloric, salty, and laden with fat. Be careful and don't be a dummy like I was.

There are several things that I now lament not doing for myself in years past as a diabetic. One of these is not starting sooner on a meticulous program of tight blood sugar control because I was trained to care for my diabetes in a program that did not stress normalizing blood glucose or doing self home blood glucose monitoring. The other is not having a high-fiber diet when I first developed diabetes. Although I am a big advocate of fiber today, and I am in very good health for a diabetic in his third decade with this disease, I wonder if having a high-fiber diet would have had any effect on lessening the severity or retarding the onset of diabetic retinopathy, the disease that caused me to become totally blind.

Fiber is important for the diabetic because, generally, blood sugar values are lower after ingesting a meal high in dietary fiber. Also, soluble fiber directly or indirectly reduces blood fat, triglyceride, which is partly responsible for heart disease and other vascular complications. One of the most difficult problems we face as diabetics is the destruction of our vascular system through the degradation of micro– and macro–blood vessel disease. This is an insidious and long-term process, aided and abetted by the diabetes itself and a myriad of other disease processes that accompany and are a part of diabetes. If one were able to prevent clogged arteries (atherosclerosis), hardening of the arteries (arteriosclerosis), and the formation of plaques of cholesterol and fatty deposits (hyper-cholesterolemia, hypertriglyceridemia), and hyperlipidemia (high blood fats), what would be the overall effect on the target organs that diabetes so ravages, such as the eyes and kidneys? There is certainly reason to speculate that a high-fiber diet may increase the possibility of reducing the severity of microangiopathy by help-ing to reduce the accumulation of fat and cholesterol within the arteries.

The incidence of diabetes seems to be quite high all over the world but in some areas, such as rural Africa, the incidence is low. Why is this? Where there is a large dietary intake of unrefined foods, fruits, and vegetables, and an almost total lack of fat, sugar, and meat, there is very little, if any, diabetes. As scientists began studying eating behavior, it was seen again and again that in areas of high dietary fiber intake, the incidence of diabetes was low. In areas where there was little dietary fiber intake, the incidence of diabetes was high. It has become alarmingly evident that Americans do not include enough fiber in their diets. During the last three decades, through commercial processing, we have lost fiber in some of our most often consumed foods, such as the husks of grains and rice and the skins of fruits and vegetables.

Fiber means plant fiber. In the natural state, all the plants we use for food have fiber that is part of the plant tissue. Dietary fibers are the nondigestible carbohydrates, including pectin, cellulose, endo-cellulose, and lignin, which make up the cell walls of plants. In the natural state, the purpose of plant fiber tissue is to help the plant to grow, to retain vital nutrients, to heal and protect the plant from damage. Fiber is found most abundantly in raw, leafy, and tough-skinned vegetables, fruits, edible seeds, nuts, and the outer layer of grains. The human digestive system does not have the essential bac-teria needed to break down fiber; it remains more or less un-changed and is passed out of the body through the gastrointestinal system. Dietary fiber has a great capacity to absorb water, which gives bulk to the system, softens the stool, and allows easy elimination through the system.

Fiber creates a feeling of fullness, thus helping to prevent overeating. This is important for the non-insulin-dependent diabetic, as this extra bulk helps to cut back on calories without making one feel hungry. Because fiber slows down the absorption of sugar through the gut, the blood sugar is evened out. For the non-insulin-dependent diabetic, this slowing down of the transfer of sugar means that a high insulin response is avoided. By avoiding the high insulin response, feelings of hunger several hours after eating are also avoided.

For the insulin-dependent diabetic, fiber helps to even out the blood sugar highs and lows that are a part of this type of diabetes by slowing the absorption of carbohydrates in the gut. For many insulin-dependent diabetics, addition of dietary fiber has the added benefit of reducing insulin requirements. I have found this to be true for myself. With the addition of twenty grams of soluble fiber and five grams of insoluble fiber per day to my diet, I have been able to reduce my insulin intake by six units per day. In addition, and very important, I have been able to maintain more normalized blood sugar values than ever before.

Soluble fiber is fiber that goes completely into solution, or completely dissolves, when added to water. Water-soluble fiber can be found in oat bran, legumes, and other vegetables, such as black-eyed peas, beans (such as lima, kidney, navy, and pinto), carrots, green peas, and corn. Broccoli, sweet potatoes, and zucchini have some soluble fiber, as do pears, bananas, oranges, apples, and prunes. Insoluble fiber is fiber that does not go into solution, or does not completely dissolve when added to water. Insoluble fiber is found in wheat bran, whole wheat, most other whole grains, and most fruits and vegetables. Insoluble fiber is important for your digestive system and may help to prevent colon cancer. Remember, water-soluble fiber is good for digestion also, but only soluble fiber can lower blood cholesterol.

To better understand solubility, as an illustrative example, picture an eight-ounce glass of water to which you have added a tablespoon of salt. When stirred, the salt dissolves and goes completely into solution, that is, salt is soluble in water. Now, picture an eight-ounce glass of water to which you have added a tablespoon of sand. When stirred, the sand is dispersed, but it will not go into solution no matter how hard you stir. Therefore, sand is insoluble in water. Insoluble fiber can be thought of in much the same way, because when stirred, it is suspended in water, but when the stirring action stops, it will fall to the bottom of the glass and remain undissolved.

Although fiber is not digested by the human body, the benefits of adding both soluble and insoluble fiber to one's diet have been well established. All fiber, whether soluble or not, when taken in by mouth, remains undigested material. When you eat a meal with fat in it, the food travels down the esophagus and into the stomach. Various enzymes do their part in the stomach to further break down the ingested food, compress and mix the food with fluid, and pass it along to the small intestine. In the small intestine, the food must be absorbed or it will do the body no good. A message is sent to the gall bladder, which is the storage bladder for bile. The liver makes bile, but it is stored in the gall bladder. The fat molecules are too large to be absorbed within the small intestine, so a message is sent to the gall bladder because help is needed to break the fat molecules into smaller and smaller pieces for eventual absorption. The gall bladder then squeezes bile out into the intestine. The bile then breaks down these large fat molecules and now you have absorption of fat by the gut. Additionally, with the absorption of fat is reabsorption of bile.

When soluble fiber is added to the diet, it forms a gel in the gut. It acts like a protective film, and as the bile breaks down the large fat molecules, the soluble fiber gel coats the large fat molecules. In this way, the fiber gel prevents the fat and bile from being absorbed through the gut. The soluble fiber gel-fat molecule-bile complex is then passed out with a bowel movement. The prevention of fat absorption by soluble fiber is why the addition of this type of fiber is so important for the diabetic. By preventing reabsorption of bile, the enterohepatic circulation (entero meaning gut, hepatic meaning liver) is broken, thus preventing bile from returning to the liver to make more cholesterol. A diet high in soluble fiber breaks a cycle that is an important step in cholesterol synthesis.

Incorporate oat bran, leafy vegetables, and fruit to your diabetic diet to help decrease your total blood cholesterol. In studies where subjects ate a bowl of oatmeal and five oat bran muffins daily, reductions in cholesterol were dramatic, up to 19 percent, but this diet has proved to be rather difficult to maintain for very long.

When shopping for products with oat bran, be sure to study carefully the level and type of oat bran contained in the product. Oats should be the first ingredient on the label. Oats and other grains contain a small amount of fat in the natural state; however, it is primarily unsaturated fat. You will want to avoid oat bran products that contain saturated or hydrogenated oils; these oils should be avoided because they may cancel out the benefit derived from the oat bran, since they raise blood cholesterol.

As a general rule, plain oatmeal and plain oat bran cereals are a better source of soluble fiber than are processed foods. Steel-cut, rolled, quick-cooking, and instant oats have the same amount of soluble fiber per gram. The finer the cut, the quicker the cereal cooks.

Oatmeal and oat bran can be used as thickeners for soups and sauces and in making breads and muffins. Other cereal products such as Cheerios and Cracklin' Oat Bran also provide the benefits of oats in the diet. Many prepared breads and crackers contain good sources of fiber through oats and whole grains.

I derive fiber from fresh fruits and vegetables and by taking supplementary fiber, both soluble and insoluble. You should consult with your doctor and dietician concerning a high-fiber diet. Fiber supplements such as Metamucil, Citrucel, and Konsil D have proved very useful to me. I hope you will investigate this area of nutrition for yourself, discuss it with your doctor, and rethink your diet in terms of including a higher fiber content. Remember that a high-fiber diet should include drinking plenty of water and fluids, also beneficial to your health. For a list of foods high in fiber, consult the government handbook *Agriculture Handbook: Composition of Foods, Raw, Processed and Prepared* (see page 190).

Let us review briefly the federal government nutritional guidelines to promote healthful eating and reduce the risk of food-related diseases within the general population. These guidelines are also part of the recommendations for principles of good nutrition by the American Diabetes Association.

1. *The diet should be varied and include all food groups.* There are fifty known nutrients that the body needs to maintain a good state of health. No single food or food group will contain all the necessary nutrients. The more varied and balanced your diet becomes, the less likely you will be to develop a deficiency or excess of any nutrient. A varied diet also reduces the risk of exposure within our food chain to contaminants, which seem to be so prevalent today.

It is important to choose food from the major food groups, milk and milk products, fruits and vegetables, bread, and meat. The new chart put out by the federal government is a pyramid that lists the following groups: fiber at the base of the pyramid, thus indicating that food high in fiber should be consumed in highest quantity, complex carbohydrates next, then proteins, then fat, and then at the tip of the pyramid, and thus indicating that this should be included in the diet in the least quantity, simple carbohydrates, sugar.

2. *In order to achieve proper weight, calorie intake and exercise should be adjusted to the individual.* Calories are the basic measurement of units of energy taken in and used up by the body. Fat is the result of eating food with more calories than the body can use, that is, unused calories are converted into fat. Fat is the main storage depot for energy. To give you an idea of the caloric requirement, in order to lose one pound of fat, you must cut 3,500 calories from your food intake. Exercise will also help in reducing fat through the utilization of these excess calories. For the diabetic, excess fat should be strictly avoided.

3. *Limit fat and consumption of high-fat foods.* Fatty foods pose more than just a weight problem. It has now been well established that fat, especially saturated fats and food high in cholesterol, are the primary contributors to heart disease and other vascular diseases. Because diabetes in and of itself accelerates these disease processes, the addition of high dietary fat makes a bad problem worse. The average American gets 40 to 50 percent of his or her total calories from fat. It is recommended that this be reduced to 30 percent of total calories.

4. *Carefully increase intake of complex carbohydrates and limit intake of simple carbohydrates.* Your intake of complex, unrefined carbohydrates should be increased, but only with the advice of your

doctor or dietician. Many diabetics make the mistake that they can eat all the complex carbohydrates they want, which is not true. The intake of simple, refined carbohydrates should be limited and carefully watched. When measured gram for gram, all carbohydrates have the same caloric value; however, different sources of carbohydrates vary in nutritional value. There are three different types of carbohydrates. These are monosaccharides, disaccharides, and polysaccharides. The simple carbohydrate, sugar, is an example of a mono- or disaccharide. Monosaccharides are sugars containing one sugar group per molecule, and disaccharides are sugars containing two sugar groups per molecule. These simple or refined carbohydrates should be limited on your diet.

Complex carbohydrates, the types that should be increased in your diet, refer to polysaccharides, which contain many sugar groups per molecule. Complex carbohydrates are found in beans, peas, grains, legumes, and vegetables. The natural sugars found in fruit and milk are examples of simple carbohydrates. When these simple carbohydrates are refined and processed into commercial sugars and other sweeteners, they retain their calories but, nutritionally speaking, the calories are "empty." As an example, if you were to eat several grams of confectioner's sugar, a refined carbohydrate, you would be taking in calories, but in terms of nutrition, you would be getting very little.

5. *Increase consumption of fiber-containing foods.* It is the opinion of many nutritionists, registered dieticians, and diet counselors that the single most important thing you can do for your health is to greatly increase your consumption of fiber. Fiber, or roughage, is the portion of a plant that the human digestive system cannot digest. Good sources of fiber include unrefined complex carbohydrates such as fresh vegetables and fruits, whole grains, peas, and beans.

6. *Reduce the intake of sodium (salt).* There has been a lot of controversy concerning high blood pressure and the intake of too much salt. Generally, Americans consume too much salt, and many manufacturers are aware of this fact and have begun to develop products with lowered sodium content. Table salt, approximately 40 percent sodium, is the main source of sodium in the American diet. Convenience foods and fast-food restaurants should be watched for the sodium content in their food products. Bacon,

pickles, canned soups, peanut butter, and salad dressings are notoriously high in sodium content. Read the package labels and choose a product that has been manufactured with low sodium content.

7. *Limit the consumption of alcohol to minimum levels, if consumed at all.* Alcohol has almost no nutritional value. It does contain calories, empty calories, that could cause you to skip a meal. If you drink, moderation is the watchword. One or two drinks per day may not harm you if you are an adult.

The concept of becoming a healthy diabetic involves more than just eating the correct items and in the correct quantities. Good health for the diabetic is a concept for living. In order to become a healthy diabetic, a meticulous program of all three of the major components of the diabetes management regime must be followed carefully, and although we all experience times when we will stray from this management program, adherence to it most of the time is in our best interest.

16

Vitamins

Vitamin and supplement intake for the diabetic is important because we lose vital nutrients due to the daily stress diabetes puts on our bodies. It is in your best interest to study this area, consult with your doctor and dietician in order to obtain their recommendations, and to better educate yourself by studying the labels on the food products you buy. Improved labeling indicates the vitamin content in a wide variety of foods today from canned goods to cereals and breads, but many foods, including fresh vegetables, fruit, fish, meat, and poultry products do not have vitamin information labeling. It is best to consult a good book on nutrition.

Over the last twenty years, nutritionists have researched the vitamins necessary to best help us live in a nearly disease-free state, thus providing the best nutrition for our brain and body. In 1958 the federal Food and Drug Administration (FDA) established the minimum daily requirements of vitamins felt to be adequate for most people. It was not long after this that these minimums were found to be entirely too low, so in 1973, the FDA introduced a new information system and labeling called the U.S. RDA Standards, or recommended daily allowances.

At about the same time as the RDAs were established by the FDA, the National Academy of Science and the National Research Council began publishing lists of vitamins known as recommended daily dietary allowances. The levels of vitamins found in these lists were about the same as the government standards but contained more precise information regarding age and sex.

I am a strong advocate for established RDAs for the betterment of our overall health. Please keep in mind, however, that these RDAs are the minimum recommendations of all the essential vitamins; the minimum of some vitamins is not nearly an optimal amount in today's world, especially when dealing with diabetes.

As an infant, my mother gave me liquid vitamins via a dropper, and as I grew up, I took One-A-Day vitamins. By the time I was in college, I was taking a combination of B-complex, lecithin, vitamin E, and an antistress formulation along with vitamin A, and multiple daily doses of vitamin C. Because I studied biochemistry as an undergraduate, I began adding more and more vitamins to my daily intake.

While still in college, I was told by a pharmacist for whom I had the greatest respect that the B vitamins were crucially important for the optimal functioning of the brain. Actually, the B vitamins are more important than any other vitamin when it comes to proper brain function. The B vitamins are not stored in the body for long periods and are called water-soluble vitamins. Therefore, these vitamins must be replenished on a daily basis. The four most important B vitamins for a healthy brain and nervous system are:

Folic acid. Folic acid, or folate, is a member of the B-complex vitamins that are necessary for the normal production of red blood cells.

Vitamin B12—Cyanacobalamin. Vitamin B12 plays an important biochemical role in the formation of the myelin sheath that surrounds the nerve fibers in the spinal cord, brain, and peripheral nerves. This vitamin can be given by injection intramuscularly and is recommended (along with folate) for the treatment of pernicious anemia.

Vitamin B1—Thiamine. This vitamin has profound implications for brain function and a deficiency may cause mental deterioration, including memory loss, numbness of the hands and feet, and abnormalities of eyeball movements.

Vitamin B6—Pyridoxine. Research on vitamin B6 indicates that this compound is crucial to the important role of metabolism of the brain. It has been determined that symptoms of low vitamin B6 levels are gastrointestinal distress and increased states of irritability.

These four B vitamins are the most important for proper brain functioning, and are therefore important for the best health of the diabetic, because diabetics suffer insulin reactions that dangerously lower the blood sugar that feeds the brain. After many years of diabetes and insulin reactions, some damage to brain cells can occur. By maintaining a daily intake of the B vitamins, some protection can be achieved to insure a healthy brain and spinal cord.

Minerals are crucial to diabetics, especially the mineral zinc, which assists the healing process. Zinc, along with most other minerals (such as copper and iodine), is usually depleted by diabetics at a much greater rate than it is absorbed into the system. This is one of the reasons that diabetics have difficulty with healing wounds. Diabetics should supplement all the essential minerals, such as zinc, selenium, copper, and manganese.

Iron levels are closely monitored on routine blood tests; levels that are too high or too low can cause serious medical implications. Iron is required by the body only in very small amounts. Iron is important for proper oxygen transfer. If the red blood cell count is found to be too low, oxygen transport becomes diminished, thereby causing less oxygen to get to the brain. This, in turn, causes fatigue, malaise, and confusion and is called iron-deficiency anemia. Usually this condition can be quickly reversed by supplementing the diet with iron, being careful not to add too much. If iron levels are too high, it could cause some malfunction to the heart.

Electrolytes are compounds that conduct an electric charge while in a solution like the blood; as this occurs, they dissociate into ions. Ions, positively or negatively charged particles, are found inside and outside the membranes of nerve cells and fibers; they may help potentiate the excitation of the nerve itself. Ion concentration in and around the nerve cell is related to the concentration of ions in the blood serum circulating around the brain. The essential ions are potassium, sodium, calcium, chloride, magnesium, and carbonate. The serum level of these ions must fall within a narrow normal range in order to avoid symptoms of brain dysfunction and illness. Your doctor will monitor these levels during routine blood testing.

It only makes good sense that we do all that is possible to maintain the highest performance of our brain, heart, liver, and kidneys. We must provide the maximum nutrition for each of these vital organs. Diabetes places unusual stress on our bodies, so it makes good sense to take vitamins and supplements that will provide maximum benefit.

I have discovered a young company in Houston, Texas, Progressive Research Labs, that is dedicated to the health of the diabetic. The owner and founder of the company is not a diabetic himself, but his father is, and the severity of his father's case inspired him to research the nutritional demands of the diabetic body. His research led him to study the metabolic effects of using chromium picolinate, chromium GTF (glucose tolerance factor), and vanadyl sulfate for diabetics and he designed a product called Diabetic Nutrition (patented in 1996) that uses these compounds (see page 181).

During the early to mid 1990s, the nutrient that was most discussed for diabetics was chromium picolinate, which was discovered and patented by the United States Department of Agriculture. Apparently, chromium plays a significant role in the metabolism of glucose. A recent study has shown a strong correlation between the deficiency of chromium and the adult onset of diabetes. The study examined borderline and Type II diabetics and found that 85 percent of these patients were grossly deficient in chromium. Chromium increases the number of insulin receptor sites and makes the receptors more sensitive to insulin. The irony is that sugar consumption depletes chromium levels in our body and when these levels are low, diabetics have difficulty metabolizing glucose.

Chromium GTF (glucose tolerance factor) is another important nutrient for diabetics. It is a niacin-bound form of chromium that is tremendously effective in regulating glucose levels and is essential for the diabetic to supplement in his dietary program.

One of the more serious aspects of diabetes is insulin resistance, the component of the disease that perpetuates it from the prediabetic state to Type I insulin dependency. It can ultimately lead to pancreatic exhaustion because insulin in the system is not being properly absorbed into the blood cell at the insulin receptor site. Thus the body sends a signal to the pancreas to produce more insulin although there really is an ample amount. This process literally wears out the pancreas by working it overtime until it gives out. The diabetic must then rely on insulin injections instead of the pancreas.

Vanadyl sulfate is a mineral that reduces insulin resistance. Many insulin-dependent diabetics have been able to significantly reduce the amount of insulin they require when using vanadyl sulfate. Vanadyl sulfate allows greater penetration of insulin into the blood cell via the insulin receptor site and because of this the insulin in the system is more efficient, so less of it is required to metabolize glucose. Vanadyl sulfate also activates glucose transport and stimulates carbohydrate uptake in the liver. It also greatly improves circulation in the diabetic. Some medical researchers are hopeful that vanadyl sulfate may well prove to be one of the most significant developments for the diabetic since the advent of insulin.

Vision Nutrition, also produced by Progressive Research Labs, uses bilberry, a compound used by the Royal Air Force during World War II to increase the visual acuity of its bomber pilots. This product also contains lutin and super antioxidants known to increase the performance of collagen-elastin fibers to strengthen the eye and other tissues.

I have used both products—Diabetic Nutrition and Vision Nutrition—in combination for almost a year now, with some very satisfying results. My energy level has increased and I find that my insulin reactions are not as severe as they were prior to my use of these products, perhaps due to the chromium.

Whatever dietary program you embark on, discuss it with your doctor. As always, remember that educating yourself, along with using common sense and balance, is always the best way to go.

17

Care of the Diabetic Foot

We take our feet for granted, with the attitude that they will always be there to get us where we need to go. Only when we feel some level of discomfort with our feet do we stop for a moment to care for them. Perhaps you may feel that because your feet are in great shape today, you have no need to be concerned about them. I know I felt that way as a teenager. Let me assure you that once you have lived with diabetes as long as I have, you will take to heart all precautions and recommendations provided to you by acknowledged experts and will take fewer chances in areas of your life that may cause complications to your diabetes.

The breakdown of the foot in the diabetic is most commonly due to a combination of factors, including neuropathy and infection, with or without some level of vascular impairment—a multitude of factors that combine to create major problems that can lead to the amputation of the foot or leg. Imagine a diabetic foot with some moderate level of vascular impairment. There may be no symptoms associated with this vascular impairment, and this condition may be fully compatible with the life expectancy of the foot. However, if an ingrown toenail or ulcer develops on the foot, and if this condition continues untreated due to lack of pain sensation (from diabetic neuropathy), the infection may spread. The infection may then become gross, demanding more of a blood supply than the blood vessels to the foot can provide. If gangrene results, an amputation may become imminent in order to save the life of the diabetic.

An infection can begin because the white cells that normally fight infection are not able to perform correctly; the levels of high blood glucose prevent them from doing so. Because bacterial pathogens and other factors are running rampant, this causes inflamed tissue, abscess formation, and occasionally blood-borne infections. The latter condition is extremely serious, and hospitalization is mandatory if the foot and the life of the diabetic are to be saved. Blood-borne infection is known as sepsis, and if you make a careful, daily examination of your feet, this should never occur. When infection runs rampant in the skin, it is known as cellulitis, and when it involves the bone, it is known as osteomyelitis, an even more serious condition.

We must accept responsibility for our feet by examining them as an everyday ritual. First, look at your nail beds and toes. Note any calluses, bunions, abrasions, nicks, or scratches. Look for signs or indications of noticeable wear, rubbing from shoes, or areas of tenderness. Check the areas above your toes for normal hair growth. Do your feet feel cold or warm? Do you have any pain when walking? Do you have signs of athlete's foot or cracking between your toes? Are your feet sensitive to hot or cold? Do you experience tingling or burning sensations in your feet? Do your ankles swell with fluid upon prolonged standing? This is the general battery of questions you must ask yourself either after bathing or showering every day or when you are ready to go to sleep every night.

It is important to do this every day, in order to become familiar with any changes and to watch for infection. Any infection for the diabetic is serious. An infection that may have started as a simple blister due to tight-fitting new shoes spells potential disaster for the diabetic. Take all bruises, scratches, nicks, abrasions, cuts, swelling, and any change in the condition of your feet as serious. This in no way means that you should panic over a scratch on the top of your foot caused by the cat playing with her catnip. It does mean that you will have to wash the scratch with a mild antibacterial soap and apply an antibacterial ointment such as bacitracin. You must watch that this scratch heals properly and that it does not become infected. If it does become infected, wash the area thoroughly with a mild solution of Phisoderm, an antibacterial soap available at your pharmacy, and warm water. Apply an antibacterial ointment, such as bacitracin, on the infected area, and apply a bandage. If this does not seem to work after a few days, consult with your doctor. Never hesitate to phone your doctor and explain the situation to him or her fully, including treatment you have done for yourself before you called.

There are other precautions you can take also. When preparing bathwater, make sure you check the temperature with your hands in order to avoid scalding your feet if the water has gotten extremely hot. Do not use hot-water bottles or heating pads at all. A hot-water bottle, a heating pad, and even an electric blanket can cause burns when set too high, and this could lead to infection. If you must sleep with an electric blanket, set the heat control on low. Also, before falling asleep, remember to turn the blanket off. If you have cold feet, consider wearing loose-fitting, comfortable socks to bed.

Diabetic neuropathy, a complication encountered in longer-term diabetes, often occurs after several years of uncontrolled high blood glucose. It decreases the diabetic's sensitivity to pain and upsets the delicate mechanisms that protect the normal foot. The purpose of pain sensation is to allow the body to use its strength to the maximum, just short of the point where pain tells us to stop. When the diabetic loses a great deal of pain sensation due to neuropathy, he has not lost the sensation of pain completely but just feels it at a different level. By the time he or she *does* feel pain, some level of damage may have been done. When the nerves of the feet are damaged, less sensory information is fed to the brain. Imagine walking barefoot on a very hot sidewalk on a summer day and not being able to know that the sidewalk is dangerously hot because of loss of sensation to hot and cold. In diabetic neuropathy, loss of sensation to sharp and dull, as well as tight and loose, as in the case with shoes, also occurs. A small pebble, a carpet tack, or a thumbtack that protrudes through the sole of the shoe could be unfelt and go unnoticed, and the damage to the foot could lead to amputation.

Nerve damage due to diabetic neuropathy can lead to weakness in the muscles of the legs and feet. Because these small muscles work together as a system, neuropathy can lead to problems in balance and stability. Associated foot problems can occur when small muscle imbalance is present. These problems include hammertoes, calluses, bunions, and other foot deformities. These foot deformities are dangerous because of their potential for causing infection.

When you visit your doctor, I suggest taking off your shoes and socks upon entering his or her examining room. This will make sure that the doctor remembers to examine your feet and talks to you about the condition of your feet. Your doctor can easily tell if you have any neuropathy by testing for reflex and sensation. The ankle-jerk reflex with preservation of the knee jerk is the classic check for neuropathy, and your doctor will undoubtedly check this reflex on you. Your doctor may also want to test your feet for the reaction to the prick of a needle in the "stocking distribution" test for sensation in the foot and leg. A tuning fork is also used to test for vibratory sensation response. There are other specialized tests that will enable your doctor to confirm the diagnosis of diabetic neuropathy. These tests include electromyography and/or nerve conduction velocity studies.

We now know that diabetes affects our blood vessels and that cigarette smoking decreases peripheral vascular blood flow. It is also well known that diabetes decreases peripheral vascular blood flow. So if you smoke and have diabetes, you are providing strong impetus for decreased peripheral vascular blood flow, with the attendant complications. Diabetes is one of the top four risk factors for premature hardening of the arteries, or atherosclerosis and arteriosclerosis, along with smoking, hypercholesterolemia, and hypertension. An endocrinologist explained to me that in the normal person, hardening of the arteries occurs from the nose to the toes. In the diabetic, hardening of the arteries occurs from the toes to the nose. Diabetics are particularly prone to narrowing of the arteries, atherosclerosis, in the extremities.

If you have poor circulation in your feet and legs, you may notice a lack of hair growth on the toes and the nails may look deformed and in generally poor condition. Your doctor may use a Doppler test for circulation or test you with a pulse volume recorder. Can poor circulation in the legs be remedied? Yes. The first remedy is to stop smoking. Exercise is the next most important remedy, followed by medication. Surgical bypass intervention may be necessary if all else fails. Here again, control of the diabetic condition is of utmost importance. Always begin by checking your blood sugar at home regularly. By doing this, both you and your doctor will know where you stand regarding your blood sugar control.

Diabetic foot ulcers are craterlike depressions that form on the skin of a diabetic. These ulcer formations can be due to neuropathy, to poor circulation, or to both conditions, and can become infected if bacteria is present. Bacterial pathogens can lead to big problems. If the bacteria is present long enough in the ulcer, it can become infected. Further infection may involve the bones of the feet, and osteomyelitis may occur. Further deterioration may lead to diabetic gangrene. This is the end stage of tissue deterioration, since the tissue bed is actually dead. The tissue here is black in color, dry or wet, and exudes pus. It must be given immediate attention. Many times, amputation is indicated when an area is gangrenous. By its very nature, gangrene is an indication of dead tissue. All possible precautions must be undertaken to prevent this end stage of tissue damage. Diabetic foot ulcers may be treated with bed rest and foot supports. A program of antibiotics should be enlisted if the ulcer is infected, along with close supervision by you and your doctor. Remember that if an infection gets out of control, it can lead to devastating consequences. Your primary goal is to avoid infection at all costs. Amputation is usually the end result of poor care and neglect by the diabetic.

David Knighton, M.D., while a medical student at Harvard during the 1970s, developed a miraculous breakthrough in the management of chronic, nonhealing wounds. With intense research into the blood's wound-healing factors, Knighton was able to isolate growth-factor proteins from blood platelets. These growth factors stimulate blood vessel formation and growth, promote scar tissue formation, and attract new skin cells. An aggressive new approach to wound healing has initiated a complete new therapy regime for those diabetics who have suffered an infection leading to an ulcer or wound that will not heal. A new biotechnology drug trademarked Procuren is what some are calling a miracle. Procuren is derived from the patient's own blood platelets, the component of the blood that helps in clot formation. Five different growth factors are stimulated to promote healing by new tissue formation in the wound. When Procuren is applied directly on the wound, it leads to faster healing and a more stable and durable tissue formation. At wound healing centers established across the country, diabetic foot ulcers, decubitus ulcers, venous stasis ulcers, and other nonhealing wounds from surgical procedures or trauma are treated in a program that is producing fantastic results. Many patients with nonhealing wounds are referred to a wound healing clinic in a last attempt to avoid amputation. It is interesting to note that 50 percent of the patients at a typical wound healing clinic are diabetics with peripheral vascular disease. It is estimated that 15 percent of diabetics across the country will develop some form of chronic, nonhealing wound such as foot and leg ulcers. This represents approximately 1.5 million diabetics who are faced with this serious problem every year. Using the wound care multidisciplinary team approach, it is hoped that the nearly sixty to seventy thousand amputations suffered by diabetics each year will be substantially reduced.

In cases of severe chronic wounds due to peripheral vascular disease, when a large blood vessel is involved, a circulatory vascular bypass may be performed. This is done to provide blood flow to an area that is nearly or completely cut off from its blood supply, and therefore its oxygen supply. If the area is hypoxic, or suffering from a lack of oxygen, and therefore preventing the wound from healing, hyperbaric oxygen therapy may be indicated. The patient breathes 100 percent oxygen while his entire body is exposed to a hyperbaric state, that is, where barometric pressures are higher than those at sea level. A physician closely supervises the patient, who is placed in a special chamber to receive the hyperbaric oxygenation therapy. The treatment can last for up to two hours, and arterial oxygen tension may rise to over 1400 mm Hg, whereas normal arterial oxygen tension is 100 mm Hg while breathing normal room air at sea level. These treatments continue every day for five days per week until the wound appears to respond. When used in a multidisciplinary approach to wound healing, hyperbaric oxygen treatments have been shown to promote infection-fighting white cells, new capillary growth, and new tissue formation.

For daily foot care, I have been very pleased with the skin tone improvement I have achieved by using two special products. The first is trade named Diabeti Derm, a deep moisturizing cream for severely dry diabetic skin. It is an advanced liposome complex cream containing urea, alpha hydroxy, and silk protein. It is non-irritating and should cause no allergic reaction. However, if you are prone to allergic skin reactions, consult with your doctor before using Diabeti Derm. I use this product on my legs, ankles, and heels, but it can be used on skin just about anywhere. The other product is Steuart's Foot Cream. This is made of natural oils, glycerin, comfrey extract, and melaleuca oil. If your feet are dry and cracked, daily use of this product may be very helpful. The comfrey extract soothes inflamed tissues and promotes healing, while the melaleuca oil is a natural antiseptic that comes from the melaleuca tree in Australia. This is an excellent cream for daily application to the feet. (For further information on these products, see Health Care Products in Other Resources.)

I also suggest you change shoes two or even three times per day. By doing this you decrease the possibility of any one pair of shoes causing irritation in the same area of the foot, thus reducing potential damage. Wear the first pair of shoes from 7 A.M. until 12 P.M., then switch to another pair from 12 P.M. until 5 P.M., and finally switch into comfortable slippers or tennis shoes until you are ready for bed. I believe this to be a good practice; once in the habit, I look forward to switching to another pair of shoes in the afternoon.

Here are more suggestions for daily care of your foot.

1. Examine your feet carefully every day. Remember, when you visit your doctor, take off your shoes and socks so that the doctor can carefully examine your feet.
2. Clean and dry your feet every day. Make sure the areas between your toes are dry.
3. Trim the toenails carefully after taking a shower or bath, when they are pliable and soft.
4. When trimming the toenails, be sure to trim straight across. Do not trim too closely. If you are visually impaired or blind, it may be best to file your nails.
5. Apply a lubricating lotion, such as lanolin or a lanolin-based product, to your feet. Avoid allowing this lotion to remain between the toes.
6. Place an absorbent powder in your shoes and socks.
7. If your feet sweat, change both shoes and socks two or even three times per day. Change socks every day at least.
8. Make sure your shoes fit correctly. If you have recently purchased a new pair of shoes and they are uncomfortable, take them to a shoe repair shop to have them mechanically broken in.
9. Exercise your feet to improve circulation.

10. Never walk barefoot.
11. Avoid extremes of cold and hot.
12. Never use tight elastic bands or garters.
13. Do not use over-the-counter foot treatments, including corn and callus removers and other remedies that use strong chemicals.
14. See your doctor and/or podiatrist immediately concerning any unusual condition you may notice with your feet.
15. And ABSOLUTELY DO NOT SMOKE! Most amputations are suffered by diabetics who smoke, and that is really sad in light of all that we now understand about smoking.

18

Dental Hygiene

Good oral hygiene for the diabetic is a subject that is rarely discussed, although it is vitally important to your total health care. If the diabetes is in poor control, the teeth, gums, and jawbone of the diabetic may suffer great deterioration. However, with good diabetic management, the diabetic's teeth and gums will be as healthy as those of the nondiabetic.

A dentist or oral surgeon looking into the mouth can discover signs of undiagnosed diabetes. For instance, dry mouth is a sign that alerts the dentist immediately to the possibility of diabetes. In the uncontrolled diabetic, the dentist may detect signs of a dry and burning mouth, inflamed and swollen membranes within the mouth, and loss of the particular cells (filiform papillae) lining the tongue. Even in the well-controlled diabetic, there are changes within the mouth, teeth, and gums.

It is important for the diabetic to realize that glucose is a nutrient to the bacteria present in the mouth. In the uncontrolled diabetic state, the presence of glucose is quite high and can, therefore, encourage additional bacteria to flourish in the mouth. Even with the higher glucose concentration found in the mouth, diabetics do not have a higher rate of cavities than their nondiabetic counterparts. In fact, insulin-dependent diabetics on carefully controlled diets show a reduced rate of cavities. Plaque formation and sugar in the diet are the major causes of dental cavities, but when these two factors are controlled, the cavity reduction is the same as in the nondiabetic. Fluoride has the same protective effect for the diabetic as the nondiabetic.

Diabetes is thought to accelerate periodontal disease due to the increased propensity for infection. The periodontal tissues are the supporting and surrounding tissues of the teeth, consisting of gingiva, periodontal ligament, and alveolar bone. The gingiva is the dense fibrous tissue that surrounds the necks of the teeth. The alveolar bone is the part of the jawbone where the alveolus, or tooth socket, is found, and the periodontal ligament is that connective-tissue ligament supporting the periodontal processes or gums. Inflammation of these tissues causes periodontal disease, and the process is initiated by bacterial formation in gingival plaque. If left unchecked, the bacterial plaque formation can cause an immunological response that leads to further deterioration of the connective-tissue fibers and periodontal ligament, loss of bone around the root of the tooth, and other destructive forces that may lead to loss of the teeth. Periodontal disease is characterized by the presence of specific bacteria. Regular dental checkups and daily meticulous cleanliness will help prevent its initiation and progression.

As always, it is imperative that your case of diabetes be under good glycemic control before your dentist begins any oral surgical procedure. Additionally, if your teeth and gums are in poor condition, with possible infection pockets, then achieving and maintaining good glycemic control is imperative. Many times, achieving near-normal blood glucose values will aid in overriding infections and bacterial overpopulation that lead to further deterioration of the teeth and gums.

I see my dentist every six months and have my teeth cleaned by the dental hygienist. I prefer to use toothpastes with baking soda. In the past, I prepared my own mixture using baking soda, salt, and hydrogen peroxide. Consult with your dentist to find out what toothpaste is best for you. I have found that brushing my teeth upon rising in the morning and before retiring at night works well for me. I use an antiseptic mouthwash—I have found Listerine to be the best—twice a day and try to floss my teeth at least once or twice a week. Most dental hygienists and dentists advise using dental floss every day. Also, I try to purchase a new toothbrush every three months, and clean it with Listerine mouthwash. At least once a week, I use an excellent electric toothbrush called Interplax. This is a Nicad battery-powered, rechargeable toothbrush with detachable brushes. It requires some technique to become accustomed to it, but once you do, you will have less plaque buildup and clean teeth and gums. Be careful not to brush too hard with the Interplax toothbrush or any other type of toothbrush. If you tend to be a hard brusher, as I am, purchase the soft-bristled brushes and try to remember to go easy on your teeth.

Schedule your dental appointments in the midmorning time frame, if possible. Doing this will afford you time to have breakfast and have taken your insulin or oral antidiabetic medication, thus preventing hypoglycemia. If you cannot get a midmorning appointment, then midafternoon is second best.

A Note of Caution

Unfortunately, today we live in a world of high infection rates. As diabetics, we know we are immunocompromised, making us more susceptible to infectious pathogens. Because the human immuno virus (HIV) poses such a great threat to us all, it is imperative that your dentist, oral hygienist, and other dental assistants practice the highest standards of precautionary techniques and meticulous cleanliness. Ask your dentist questions concerning practices in avoiding contracting HIV from patients and his or her practices to avoid infecting patients by either patient-to-patient contact or doctor-to-patient contact. Ask what defense he or she has installed to prevent aerosolized matter from drilling of teeth or cleaning of teeth and mucous membranes. Lastly, make sure your dentist wears the latest latex gloves and that suctioning equipment does not retain backflow from the last patient. We must remain dauntless as advocates of our health as diabetics and strive for the best care, both from ourselves and from our practitioners.

19

Male Baldness

In order to stay and remain in the best shape possible, diabetics must work a little harder, become more disciplined and meticulous, and do things a little better than those around us. Our appearance is also important, and in order to not only look our best, but to be as successful as possible, we must do all that we can to possess a confident and powerful image. Hair is a vital aspect of our overall appearance and can indeed indicate to our doctors the level of our health. Malnutrition and improper diet will eventually show up in the unhealthy texture and quality of our hair.

Hair loss is not dependent upon our station in life, race, or age. Male-pattern baldness begins in the twenties, and we can become aware of our receding hairline at an even earlier age, depending upon our own particular genetic makeup. According to one hair-transplant specialist, if we live long enough, all of us will eventually become bald. The one thing we know for sure is that hair loss can be devastating to our self-esteem and our level of confidence.

Hair transplants are the ultimate answer to replacing hair lost to aging and the balding process. To determine if this is a suitable procedure for the diabetic, I decided to investigate the procedure on myself by going in for consultations with leading hair-transplant specialists and then having the procedure performed.

First, let's review some tips that take a common-sense approach to taking the best care of the hair we have. These tips will hopefully prolong the life of your hair.

1. Do not dry your hair with an excessively hot hair dryer. In the hurry-up mode in which we often operate, it seems like the few minutes it takes to dry our hair after shampooing each morning can

be speeded up by using high heat or holding the unit too close to the head. The best practice is to use a lower heat setting and hold the unit some distance from the hair.

2. When showering, do not allow the stream of water to blast down directly on the back of your head. Showering in this manner will eventually, over a number of years, wear down the hair and help cause premature balding in the back of the head.

3. Use of a mild shampoo is best, unless you have an unusually oily scalp condition. I have found Progaine, manufactured by Upjohn of Kalamazoo, Michigan, to be very good. This shampoo adds volume and body to your hair and is excellent whether used in conjunction with Rogaine or not.

4. When towel drying, stroke upward rather than downward. Over a period of many years, the daily downward strokes we use to dry our hair slowly pull at the hairline. Using an upward stroke motion promotes the areas with abundant hair, the sides and back, toward the top of the head.

5. When brushing the hair, be gentle. Mechanical breakage of hair results in damage that can be unnecessary.

6. Ask your doctor or dietician about the advisability of using specially formulated vitamins for the hair. I use Vitamins for Hair Care, available from Nutrition Headquarters, Inc. (see Other Resources, page 180).

Hair transplant surgery has been an accepted procedure for almost forty years and has benefited from advances in microsurgical techniques. Many patients who had hair transplants years ago still have the strongly growing transplanted hair today.

There are two main procedures in hair transplant surgery: 1. micro- and minigrafts, and 2. scalp reduction. Micro- and minigrafts are made up of strips of donor hair taken from the back or sides of the scalp and cut into grafts that range in size from one to eight hairs or more, depending upon the surgeon's technique. These grafts are then transplanted into areas of the scalp where the hair is thinning. The technique itself and the artistry of the surgeon's skill have greatly advanced from methods used even five years ago. However, no federal or state agency regulates or sets minimum standards for hair transplantation. A licensed physician, even without surgical experience, can perform hair transplants, so it is important to know that the surgeon you choose is competent and has satisfied patients with his or her technique.

I spoke with Dr. Karin Montero, a gifted reconstructive and cosmetic surgeon in Austin, Texas, concerning baldness, hair transplants, and the scalp reduction technique. Dr. Montero's approach was one of sensitivity to the process of male-pattern baldness. Her philosophy is that balding is a natural process and that bald men are handsome. Only when the baldness becomes an emotional issue for the patient or when baldness is inappropriate due to age or accident should a surgical procedure become necessary. Scalp reduction is just that: the balding area of the scalp is surgically cut away. This major surgery requires a balloon inserted into each temple area for a period of three months. The balloons stretch the scalp in the areas where there is usually more hair. Once the scalp has been stretched, the balding area is excised and the flaps sewn together. Micro- and minigrafts are then used to soften the look and create a full head of hair. This procedure is for the severely bald man who wishes to reverse his looks and is willing to spend a great deal of time and money to correct the problem.

Another alternative is an artificial hairpiece made of either synthetic fiber or human hair. Most hairpieces attach to the scalp with glue. One method of attachment unsuitable for the diabetic uses wire loops surgically implanted into the scalp; these can cause serious infection because the holes in the scalp never fully heal. One of the newer attachment techniques is called tunnel grafting. In this procedure, grafts of skin taken either from the groin area or from behind the ear are surgically excised and grafted onto the scalp. This forms living loops; when fully healed, they can accept plastic fasteners that attach to the hairpiece. Due to possible infections, this is also not an appropriate procedure for the diabetic. In the hair-weaving technique, the hairpiece is attached to and woven into the hair already on the scalp. As your hair grows, the hairpiece becomes loose; every two months the hair must be cut and the hairpiece reattached. A drawback to this procedure is possible damage to the natural hair.

Most manufacturers suggest two hairpieces be purchased to allow one piece to be cleaned while the other is worn. Those men with hairpieces to whom I have spoken have cautioned against wearing the hairpiece during showering and swimming. The newer hairpieces may allow for this activity; however, damage to the hairpiece may occur. The scalp is part of the skin, the largest organ system of the body, and it is dynamic in its function of living and "breathing." If you bond the hairpiece with a strong adhesive for long periods, then the living and breathing aspects of the scalp tissue will be affected. The diabetic must be especially careful in dealing with a hairpiece; cleanliness and avoiding infections are very important.

Hair Enhancers

Back in the early 1980s, I tried a product called New Generation, consisting of a two-part system of shampoo with a conditioner that was placed on the scalp after shampooing. Although this company could not legally claim actual regrowth of hair, I used this combination for many years, until I switched over to Rogaine, and I found the New Generation products to be helpful in the early stages of my hair loss.

The federal Food and Drug Administration, FDA, prohibits the manufacturer of any hair-enhancing formulation to use wording in their advertising promising that their product will definitely grow hair, with the exception of Upjohn Pharmaceutical's Rogaine. The FDA wording is specific: "Nothing done to the hair shaft, once it emerges from the surface of the scalp, will influence hair growth." Any lotion or cream designed to influence hair growth would have to work on the hair root. Minoxidil, trade named Rogaine, is the only substance ever approved by the FDA and scientifically proven to grow hair on the scalp. It was available by prescription only until 1996, when the FDA granted it over-the-counter status.

The early studies on minoxidil began in 1980, at Harvard Medical School, where it was applied topically to treat male baldness. Thirty-five hundred men participated in their extensive testing program, and in a four-month testing period, it was found that men using Rogaine grew significantly more hair than those on placebo. In other tests Upjohn found that after twelve months of using Rogaine, approximately 66 percent of the men showed either no growth or grew fine, babylike peach-fuzz hair. The final 33 percent grew moderate to dense amounts of what was termed *cosmetically significant hair*. Only about 5 percent of the men tested showed dense hair growth. Also, the men who will most significantly improve with the use of Rogaine are men in their twenties and thirties who have been balding for fewer than ten years, whose bald spot at the top of the head is less than four inches across, and who have fine hair remaining. Minoxidil has not been shown to regenerate hair along the frontal hairline, so frontal baldness is not affected.

Minoxidil was originally designed as a heart medication, so it is important for the diabetic to discuss using Rogaine with a doctor, even though it is now available as an over-the-counter product. I have used Rogaine for more than five years, and I can report only minimal regrowth of hair, but I have retained the hair I had. Certainly, it has retarded the balding process and has not adversely affected either my diabetes or my antihypertensive medication, captopril (Capoten). Rogaine must be applied topically to the scalp two times per day. An eyedropper applicator is provided with the bottle of liquid Rogaine. It is important to make sure the liquid goes directly onto the scalp and is not diverted by strands of hair. I have become comfortable in using Rogaine on a daily basis and must say that I have been very happy with the results, but remember, Rogaine must be used on an uninterrupted basis for life. If you stop using Rogaine, you will lose all the hair you gained by using it.

More on Hair Transplants

Strip grafts and flap rotation are two additional techniques that surgeons use to replace lost hair. These involve major surgery and are probably not advisable for the diabetic. In these procedures, long sections of hair are surgically removed from the back or sides of the scalp. These sections are then placed onto the balding areas of the top or front of the head to create new growth areas.

There are several problems with these procedures, including the possibility of serious infection and tissue death, causing permanent loss of the hair and scarring. An unnatural look may result if hairs grow in the opposite direction of the hairs surrounding them. These procedures require the talents of an especially gifted surgeon.

The micrograft technique is most probably the best choice for a diabetic considering undergoing this procedure. The graft is taken from the back and sides of the head, where hair is genetically pro-grammed to last a lifetime. Grafts of from two to thirty hairs are taken and then relocated to areas of thinning or balding. Termed the punch autograft technique, it is the most widely accepted and best approach for the majority of men with male-pattern baldness. After transplantation, the grafts quickly take root, followed by a short resting phase of no growth. They then begin regrowth and continue to grow for a lifetime. The hair restoration specialist/cosmetic surgeon must possess a high degree of artistic ability and must know innately what looks good. The aim of all cosmetic sur-gery is to operate on an individual and leave no trace of tampering with that person's features. A look that is natural, yet seeks the intended improvement, is the overall goal.

I had a consultation with Dr. Lee Laris of the Medical Hair Restoration Group, headquartered in Tampa, Florida, with offices in major cities. Their surgeons must first be board certified in der-matology or cosmetic surgery, then undergo an eighteen-month fel-lowship presided over by Dr. Matt Levitt, founder. I found Dr. Laris to be another example of an extremely gifted surgeon with a high degree of artistic talent. Interested in my case of long-term diabetes, he discussed my case with compassion and had no doubts concerning the success he could attain for me. I would require approximately four hundred grafts, and this could be done in a stepwise approach, with two hundred grafts per session. He explained that a complete blood chemistry along with a fasting blood glucose and a test for HIV would be necessary to get started. Prednisone, an anti-inflammatory steroid, would be ordered after the transplant session, along with a regimen of antibiotics to pre-vent any possible infection. High blood sugars can result from tak-ing prednisone, so checking your blood sugar three or four times per day is a good idea in order to stay in good control.

After making sure my blood sugar was in good control, I reported to the office of Medical Hair Restoration. Dr. Laris first removed a strip of donor hair from the back of my head that mea-sured approximately one-half inch by six inches. This area was sutured together while the assistants prepared the donor grafts. Dr. Laris then began the procedure of strategically placing the punch incisions where the donor grafts would be placed. He made 250 of these incisions and then carefully placed the donor hair shafts and follicles into the incisions. The incisions were more like tiny holes and no pain was felt since lidocaine was given locally to both the donor strip area and the top of the head where the grafts were to be placed.

Dr. Laris told me that each donor graft held between one and seven hairs. After the procedure, he carefully wrapped my entire head in gauze; I looked like I had on a turban. That night and for the next four nights I slept at a forty-five-degree angle in order to prevent swelling. Only light exercise should be engaged in during the week before the surgery. After the surgery, no exercise for a week is a good rule, as well as no sexual activity and only light physical work.

I was given prednisone as an anti-inflammatory agent to prevent swelling. I tested my blood sugar every one to two hours in order to stay in good control. I gave myself extra amounts of regular insulin in order to reduce the high blood sugars I was experiencing due to the prednisone. You must take prednisone for four or five days, so you must be diligent in maintaining good blood glucose control. You will also be applying a light coating of antibacterial ointment to the graft areas and a special application of saltwater-soaked gauze to the surgical area for five minutes, five times per day, for five days. This procedure ensures smooth skin healing of the graft area.

You will be told to carefully watch for infection and to wash your hair daily using a washcloth to prevent forceful blasts from the showerhead. The day following surgery, I went back to Dr. Laris's office to have my hair washed by one of the surgical assistants and was given more instructions as to the care of my new grafts. About ten days later I went back to have the sutures removed from the donor area in back of my head.

I have now undergone two of these procedures and have not had any difficulty in either session. Dr. Laris and his staff could not have treated me any better and I knew I was in the fine hands of a true expert.

I am extremely proud of the new hair I now have. I was not totally bald, but the frontal hair was thinning and eroding so fast that it would not have been much longer before I would have been completely bald on top. My hairline has been restored appropriately for a man in his forties, a touch a truly gifted and artistic surgeon like Dr. Laris can do so easily and professionally.

This procedure has greatly improved my self-confidence and appearance. If you are a diabetic man with thinning hair and are considering hair transplants, a discussion with your doctor is in order. Your blood sugar must be in good control in order for the grafts to continue to survive. Make sure you check your blood glucose and pay close attention to the areas from which the grafts were taken. Your hair transplant specialist will advise you of the special protocol required after the surgical procedure, and the protocol must be adhered to closely for best results.

Guidelines for Choosing a Cosmetic Surgeon

Dr. Richard Aronson, founder and past president of the American Academy of Cosmetic Surgery, suggests this list of guidelines for choosing any cosmetic surgeon:

1. Make sure, when calling for information, that you are given the name of the surgeon you will be seeing.
2. Make sure you actually have a consultation with the surgeon, not with a layperson consultant.
3. Make sure the surgeon's qualifications are readily available at the office or clinic you are visiting.
4. Fees should not be quoted over the phone, due to the fact that a qualified cosmetic surgeon can determine fees only on an individual basis during a personal consultation.
5. Make sure the surgeon spends enough time answering all of your questions in order to determine your expectations for improvement.
6. Should both you and the surgeon proceed, make sure you have a clear understanding of what to expect in terms of ultimate self-improvement, inconvenience, and cost.
7. Make sure medical photographs are taken before and after surgery so that a clear picture of the exact degree of improvement is seen following surgery.
8. Make sure the surgeon never pressures you into taking any elective surgery for which you have doubts.
9. Make sure your surgical fee includes meticulous follow-up appointments, including a series of progress checks.

20

Erectile Dysfunction in the Diabetic Male

As a healthy diabetic male with a normal sex life, discussing male erectile dysfunction may be difficult for you, or it may not be of concern to you at this time, in which case you can save this chapter for future reference. If, however, this is an area of concern for you, a consultation with your doctor would be the next step. I also suggest you read the comments by Dr. Kenneth A. Goldberg of the Male Health Clinic, Dallas, Texas in Appendix A (page 174).

Sexual wellness is moving ahead to the forefront as a key indicator of a man's total health. With our lifetimes extended and better medical, pharmaceutical, and surgical techniques being developed on a daily basis, a healthy sex life into the advanced years is entirely possible.

Erectile dysfunction is often called the most common untreated medical disorder known, and this is true all over the world. In the past, due to the difficulty in discussing this problem with his sexual partner and even his physician, a man would probably have been told to just live with it. The good news today is that most cases are easily treatable, the level of understanding has vastly improved, and male sexuality is a subject we can talk about in real terms.

In the United States, experts estimate there are thirty to forty million men who suffer erectile dysfunction or what was once medically termed impotence. It has been further estimated that fewer than 5 percent have been treated, with most men not willing to admit to erectile dysfunction, thus giving in to abstinence.

There is an abundance of information to suggest that erectile dysfunction is related to diabetes per se. There is a 50 percent reported incidence of erectile dysfunction among diabetic men, and research indicates that the figures may be above 60 percent. For diabetics, it may occur any time after adolescence; if the nerves leading to the penis that cause an erection are damaged from neuropathy, then there will be no erection. However, not all diabetics develop erectile dysfunction and not all erectile dysfunction in the diabetic is due to the diabetic condition.

Defined medically, erectile dysfunction is the chronic or persistent inability to achieve and maintain an erection satisfactory to complete sexual intercourse. What this actually boils down to is the failure of the penis to become and remain erect, in other words, erectile failure. If a man's erection is no longer firm enough or cannot last long enough to allow vaginal penetration, or if the penis loses strength upon penetration, then this constitutes an erectile dysfunction problem. When this problem becomes persistent, medical consultation is the next step, along with education as to the current therapeutic avenues. It is important to realize that a combination of factors, including erotic brain stimulus, a healthy vascular system, undamaged nerves, and adequate hormones are all necessary for a normal erection. When any one of these processes is affected by injury, disease, or a host of psychological factors, the result may be erectile dysfunction.

Many men are surprised to learn that erectile dysfunction is not a normal consequence of aging. Yes, there are changes in erectile function as we age, and as a man grows older, additional stimulus is needed to produce an erection. As we age, the erection is harder to maintain, less rigid, and certainly more vulnerable to emotional factors. However, a healthy man who maintains a healthy sexual interest and desire, and who has an interested and willing partner, should expect to have usable erections once or twice a week well into his eighties.

The Penis

Consisting of three parallel cylinders made up of spongy tissue and bound in thick membranous sheets, the penis is a wondrous organ in both its form and function. The spongy body is the corpus spongeosum and is the cylindrical body on the underside of the penis. With the dual purpose of carrying both urine and semen, the urethra runs through the middle of the spongy body and exits at the tip of the penis via the urethra meatus, or the urinary opening. The spongy body on the underside of the penis appears as and feels like a straight ridge. The cavernous bodies, corpora cavernosa, are the other two cylinders of the penis. These are positioned above the spongy body and are aligned side by side. These three cylinders all consist of irregular, spongelike tissue and are lined with small blood vessels. During the time of sexual arousal, this tissue, covered by an elastic tissue tunic, swells with blood, thus producing an erection.

The cavernous bodies, corpora cavernosa, extend through the entire length of the penis. They meet at the coronal ridge, where the glans penis is the tip or distal end of the penis. The urethra forms its opening at the glans penis and extends through the penis into the bladder.

Internally, and past the point where the penis is attached to the body, the cavernous bodies branch apart to form tips that are firmly attached to the pelvic bones. Both inside and apart from the cylindrical bodies, the penis has many blood vessels and a pattern of veins can be seen on the outer skin of the erect penis. The penis is also highly innervated, making it very sensitive to pressure, touch, and temperature. Consisting entirely of corpus spongeosum, the tip of the penis (the glans or head) has a higher concentration of sensory nerve endings than does the shaft. Thus, the head of the penis is particularly sensitive to physical stimulation.

The foreskin, or prepuce, of the glans is formed of the freely movable skin covering the shaft of the penis. Newborn males are usually circumcised, and this procedure, circumcision, is the surgical removal of the foreskin. This minor surgical procedure is usually performed after birth and results in the glans of the penis being fully exposed at all times.

Dr. Kenneth A. Goldberg (please see his comments on page 174), informed me of the latest thinking about erectile function according to the National Institutes of Health position paper and the current understanding within urological research. Erections occur when nerves are influenced by the brain sending a message down to the penis. In the brain, chemical neurotransmitters are released that cause the spongy tissue of the penis to relax and allow blood to flow in. There is a passive compression of the veins leading to the trapping of blood, producing an erection.

In the male diabetic, a number of pathological processes can occur, including impaired blood flow, loss of sensation that sends messages back to the brain, loss or damage to nerves sending messages from the brain to the penis, potential damage to neurotransmitters, and, finally, damage to the blood vessels' spongy tissue, which can lead to problems with trapping of the blood.

Dr. Goldberg also stated that erections go away because the neurotransmitter norepinephrine is released, which causes vasoconstriction (blood vessel tightening), thereby allowing the blood to leave the penis. This is what occurs during anxiety, when adrenaline is secreted. It is important to remember that erection is but one component of the sexual act. Orgasm and ejaculation are two different phases and one can get any component without the other.

The Scrotum and Testicles

The scrotum consists of a thin, loose sack of skin that is beneath the penis and contains the testicles or testes. Sperm production occurs in the testes and is dependent on a stable temperature. The scrotum is able to maintain a stable temperature due to a layer of muscle fibers lining the sack. These muscle fibers contract involuntarily in response to cold, exercise, or sexual stimulation. This action causes the testicles to be drawn up against the body. During hot weather, the scrotum relaxes, allowing the testicles to hang more freely and away from the body. The male gonads are called the testes or testicles. The two testes, contained in the scrotum, are approximately equal in size, with one testicle usually hanging slightly lower than the other. Being extremely sensitive to touch and pressure, the function of the testes is for hormone and sperm production.

Testosterone is a male hormone produced by Leydig cells within the testes. It is responsible for male sexual development and plays an important part in sexual interest and function. Sperm is manufactured in the seminiferous tubules. The seminiferous tubules are incredibly small, tightly coiled tubules that, if laid out end to end, measure over one-quarter mile (about five hundred meters) in length. The process of sperm production requires sixty days; sperm is in a constant state of production from puberty forward, with billions of sperm produced every year.

The seminiferous tubules empty into the epididymis, an intricate network of highly coiled tubules that are folded against the back side of each testicle. It is within the epididymis that the sperm cells spend several weeks traveling as they reach their fully mature state. Next, the sperm are carried into the vas deferens, long tubes (sixteen inches or about forty centimeters) that leave the scrotum and curve alongside and behind the bladder. The prostate gland is a walnut-sized gland that has a muscular portion and a glandular portion. Surrounding the urethra, the prostate is located directly below the bladder. The relationship between the prostate and the urethra can be likened to a ball (the prostate) through which a string (the urethra) passes.

It is important to have regular prostate examinations performed by your physician, especially after the age of forty. Your doctor will examine your prostate for signs of cancer or infection. The prostate is responsible for producing 30 percent of the seminal fluid (of which 5 percent is sperm), which is the fluid that is expelled from the penis during ejaculation. The seminal vesicles produce the other 70 percent of seminal fluid. The seminal vesicles lie against the back of the base portion of the bladder and join with the ends of the vas deferens to form the ejaculatory ducts. These ejaculatory ducts join the urethra, which creates the pipeline to the end of the penis.

The physiology of human sexual arousal is the cornerstone of the procreation of our species. A better understanding of the functions involved in male sexual physiology resulted in the late 1960s when pioneers William H. Masters and Virginia E. Johnson began research on human subjects. Their exhaustive study evaluated sexual parameters in a large sample of men and women. Their book, *Human Sexuality,* published in 1966, is the textbook for college and graduate-level courses on human sexual behavior.

The Male Orgasm

Occurring in two distinct stages, the orgasm of the male is unlike that found in females. The vas deferens, the two tubes that carry sperm, and the prostate and seminal vesicles are involved in the first stage of male orgasm. Contractions in these two areas force semen into the bulb of the urethra, leading to ejaculation. Before the actual ejaculatory response, there is a period of ejaculatory inevitability. This phase is a feeling of having reached the brink of control, as the actual contractions begin. Losing control, as it were, is actually quite accurate because at this point ejaculation cannot be prevented.

In the second stage of male orgasm, contractions of the prostate gland combined with contractions of the urethra and penis cause ejaculation, the delivery of sperm out of the penis. Sperm does not appear at the tip of the penis until several seconds have elapsed after ejaculatory inevitability.

The neck of the urinary bladder is tightly closed during ejaculation to prevent mixing of urine and semen. Semen is propelled forward by rhythmic contractions of the prostate, perineal muscles, and shaft of the penis, which all help to create the physical force required for the ejaculatory propulsion of semen out of the penis.

Male orgasm and ejaculation are not the same process; however, they occur simultaneously in most men under normal circumstances. Orgasm is defined as the acme or climax of the sexual act and involves the sudden rhythmic contractions, in the pelvic region and elsewhere in the body, that release sexual tension along with the mental sensation that coincides with this experience, whereas ejaculation refers strictly to the release of semen, accompanied by orgasm or not.

Retrograde Ejaculation

Retrograde ejaculation is a sexual problem found in some diabetic men due to diabetic neuropathy. There is an involvement of the pelvic autonomic nervous system that involves both emission, which is the delivery of the seminal fluid into the urethra, and ejaculation, which is the forceful propulsion of the fluid from the urethra to the outside. In long-term or poorly controlled diabetes, neuropathy impairs the pelvic autonomic nerves and the internal vesicle sphincter. In this situation, the neck of the bladder does not close off properly during orgasm, with the result of the semen being propelled backward into the bladder. There are no harmful effects, but infertility can result and there may be some loss of sensation, along with slight mental anguish at the loss of production of semen at climax.

Problems of fertility and sterility must be considered if retrograde ejaculation is diagnosed in the diabetic male. There are techniques available today whereby the sperm is captured in the bladder. Once captured, sperm is spun in a centrifuge, washed, and then either used in artificial insemination or with in vitro fertilization.

The Causes of Sexual Dysfunction

Medical literature classifies the causes of sexual dysfunction as either organic or psychosocial. In organic sexual dysfunction, medical or physical causes include illness, drug effects or addiction, and injury. Psychosocial factors include psychological effects, interpersonal attitudes, cultural factors, and environmental factors. It has been pointed out by many sexologists that sexual dysfunction may result from a combination of organic and psychosocial factors. It has been estimated that up to 90 percent of all sexual dysfunction is organic in nature. In 10 to 15 percent of cases, sexual difficulty is worsened by psychological factors although they may not be the sole cause.

Erectile Dysfunction

Vascular disease and diabetes are the two major organic causes of erectile dysfunction. It is important to realize that although alcoholism can lead to damaged nerves, which can then cause erectile dysfunction, it is not as prominent a cause as other problems, such as vascular disease, faced by the diabetic. So if you have diabetes and drink too much alcohol, you will most probably have problems in achieving an erection. Other causes of erectile dysfunction are injury, circulatory problems, hormone deficiencies, and certain prescription medications (antihypertensive medications) and street drugs (amphetamines, barbiturates, and narcotics).

It is very important for men to realize that an erection is not an immediate "on demand" response, just as the fact that we are unable to cause our blood pressure to drop or to lower our pulse rate on demand. Natural reflexes that produce the response necessary for an erection can take over when the fear of performance is removed or reduced substantially. Erections come and go naturally, so the tendency to rush sexual engagement when an erection is produced, fearing that it will go away and not return, should be avoided. The rush to sexual performance is another form of performance anxiety, and the usual result is loss of erection, caused by adrenaline.

Premature Ejaculation

Premature ejaculation is not related to an organic dysfunction. Men who experience this problem cannot exert voluntary control over ejaculation and, once sexually aroused, ejaculate quickly and cannot resume intercourse for an undetermined period of time. Premature ejaculations often occur with little direct penile stimulation. Diabetes plays no causative role in premature ejaculation, and most men pass through some phase of this problem at some time of their life. Doctors now use the antidepressant drugs anafronil, Zoloft, and Prozac to retard ejaculation. There are a number of good books on this subject (see Bibliography, page 193).

Restoring Erectile Function

A great deal of the present-day research into psychosocial causes of erectile dysfunction indicates that there are associations between sexual dysfunction and developmental traumas, psychological traits, relationship difficulties, and behavior patterns. Unfortunately, research into this area cannot prove what causes the sexual dysfunction. Many men with disastrous psychosocial backgrounds have an entirely normal sex life. Conversely, others with a normal psychosocial background may have some degree of, or even complete, sexual dysfunction. Today, there exists a great debate as to what percentage of men suffers from a psychological rather than physical basis of erectile dysfunction. The pendulum has now swung from the pioneering work done by Masters and Johnson, who said that 90 percent of men suffer dysfunction due to psychological problems, to the current data, which says that 90 percent are due to a physical basis.

Developmental factors involved in psychosocial sexual dysfunction include the child who was brought up feeling that sex is sinful, shameful, and/or dirty, or the child who was severely and repeatedly punished for touching his sexual parts or for talking about or engaging in childlike sex play. In these situations, the child grows up with a distorted view of sex, with the result that sex is unpleasurable and unhealthy. Intensive research into this area now indicates that many men with sexual dysfunction have normal personalities, with no signs of emotional illness or distress, and therefore it is with great difficulty that the practitioner tries to find an answer to the primary cause of the sexual dysfunction. If you have diabetes, then this causative factor must be fully explored in order to ascertain if it is some aspect of the diabetic state that is causing erectile dysfunction. A patient and understanding medical team must be utilized in order to obtain the best results and restore sexual function.

There has been a great deal of innovative research into restoring penile function to men with varying levels of erectile dysfunction, so much so that there is available some form of restorative treatment for almost all men who suffer erectile dysfunction.

Because the nerves and blood vessels are so vitally important to erectile function, it only makes good sense that good blood sugar control will improve performance in this area. If we keep our blood sugar in tight control, we place less stress on our nervous system and vascular system. The best way to avoid complications of diabetes is to maintain strict blood glucose control, a healthy diet, and vigorous daily exercise.

Topical Medications

The topical drugs minoxidil, nitroglycerine, and other topical vasodilators have not, at this time, been adequately studied for their effectiveness. Your doctor must teach you how to apply one of these drugs directly onto the penis. These agents open up the blood vessels and thereby increase blood flow, facilitating an erection. A condom must always be worn; otherwise the sexual partner may experience side effects such as severe headache and stomach upset. More research looms in the future for topically applied vasodilators.

Oral Medications

Oral medications such as yohimbine and trazadone must be taken on a daily basis and usually require six to eight weeks before any noticeable improvement results. Dosages of these medications will vary and must be determined by your doctor. Yohimbine HCl therapy frequently improves sexual desire, and 30–40 percent of patients report improved erections. Effectiveness of this drug is highest when the erectile dysfunction is psychological or of unknown cause. The effectiveness of yohimbine is enhanced when used with trazadone. Reported side effects include mild dizziness, nausea, nervousness, and headache. Trazadone is an antidepressant and has not formally been studied as a treatment for erectile dysfunction. However, taken daily in combination with yohimbine, it may improve the quality of erections in 25 percent of patients.

A new oral medication on the horizon is sildenafil, a phosphodiesterase inhibitor, which has been studied in Europe and is beginning to be studied in the United States. Success has been good, especially for men who do not have significant vascular impairment or obstruction of their tissue.

Hormonal Treatment

Testosterone is the predominant male hormone; estrogen is the predominant female hormone. Testosterone replacement therapy seems to improve erectile function only in those men who are severely deficient in testosterone level. It is rarely helpful in those whose testosterone is within normal limits. It is given by injection either on a monthly or bimonthly protocol. Your primary-care physician may want you to be seen by an endocrinologist in order that your testosterone levels can be carefully monitored and your success in using this treatment can be carefully evaluated. Too much testosterone can stimulate growth of prostatic tissue, cause liver damage and tumors, stop sperm production, and increase fluid retention. This hormone should be administered with extreme caution in those who have a history of prostate cancer or heart, kidney, or liver disease. Testosterone transdermal patches are now available for use in testosterone replacement therapy. These patches can be placed on the scrotum or elsewhere on the body. A lifelong dependency can develop when using testosterone replacement therapy, and in severe cases, testicular atrophy can occur.

Penile Implants

This is a surgical procedure and will require a good deal of study on your part and consultation with your doctor before a decision can be made as to whether this is right for you. Your sexual partner should be brought along for each stage of the explanations, from initial consultation to final decision.

I have spoken to several men who have undergone penile implant surgery, and most are amazed at the level of pain involved with the procedure. Most told me that they were not initially prepared for the discomfort they experienced, but were happy with the final results. There are a host of complications that can occur with penile implants. For diabetics, infection can be very serious, so your doctor will be maintaining a close watch on your daily progress.

The penile prosthesis is a fixed or mechanical device surgically implanted into the two corpora cavernosa of the penis. This allows for an erection suitable for intercourse as often as desired, without affecting sensation, ejaculation, or orgasm. Penile implants come in two basic types. The simpler of the two types is a pair of fixed, semirigid, malleable, silicone-covered rods that are implanted inside the shaft of the penis. When these rods were first developed, users complained of having to deal with a permanent state of partial erection that caused embarrassment. Refinement to these rods includes a bendable wire core, which enables the user to allow the partially erect penis to be bent down against the inner thigh. This enables the man to be comfortable when dressed in close-fitting clothing. Protrusion of the rods through the glans of the penis and poor erection may result if sizing is incorrect.

The inflatable pump device is much more complicated and expensive and therefore requires a great deal of commitment of time, money, and the learning process. There are three basic types, all of which may be subject to mechanical failure.

1. The multicomponent prosthesis consisting of a fluid pump located in the scrotum, a reservoir located in the abdomen, and two inflatable cylinders.

2. A self-contained inflatable prosthesis composed of two sealed cylinders, each containing fluid, a pumping mechanism, and a release valve. About 5 percent undergo mechanical failure within five years.

3. A self-contained mechanical implant device made of an intricate series of interlocking plastic blocks, with a spring-loaded steel

cable passing through them. This system is not difficult to operate. However, mechanical failure can still occur.

In the surgical procedure, two tapered inflatable cylinders are implanted in the penis. These cylinders are connected by a system of tubing that goes to a reservoir containing fluid used to fill the cylinders in the shaft of the penis. The fluid-containing reservoir system is implanted in the lower abdomen. Fluid is moved into the cylinders by pinching a single pump and valve located in the scrotum. As the fluid moves into the cylinders, a natural-looking erection is produced. When the valve is released, the fluid moves out of the cylinders and back into the reservoir, and the penis is returned to the flaccid state.

Penile implant surgery is indicated when erectile dysfunction is so severe that no other means will produce an erection. Some men have complained of the artificial nature of the penile implants. However, when the man and his sexual partner become accustomed to its use, a great deal of pleasure can be achieved, in terms of both sexual satisfaction and the emotional security of having one's "manhood" regained.

It is imperative that you understand that penile implants can cause complications. Furthermore, because they are mechanical devices, some technical difficulties may be present. Some of the early studies noted that infections and mechanical problems developed in 40 percent of implant cases. This usually required removal of the device or a repeat surgical implant in order to correct the problem. Newer studies indicate that mechanical failure results in 5–10 percent of cases and infection in 3–5 percent of cases; this may result in removal or replacement of the prosthesis. It is important to understand that the surgical placement of any kind of prosthesis permanently alters the internal structure of the penis; natural erections will rarely, if ever, return.

Penile revascularization and venous ligation are surgical procedures that are very complex, so much so that they can be likened to a heart bypass operation, although these procedures do not carry the same amount of risk to the patient. Only a very few patients are appropriate candidates for this type of procedure, about one case in one hundred; of these, the success rate is only 20–30 percent. Postoperatively, six weeks is required before attempting intercourse. The relapse rate is very high, about two years; two years of erectile function may or may not be suitable for you. Infection may occur and numbness may persist near the incision site, which means limited penile sensation. These procedures are available at only a few select medical centers in the United States. Due to the risks, I would not suggest this type of surgical procedure for the diabetic at the present time. As these procedures become technically advanced, perhaps they will offer a new frontier in vascular revitalization of the penis.

External Vacuum Therapy

External vacuum therapy, available since about 1973, is the least invasive of the erectile dysfunction therapies and constitutes the first line of therapy for erectile dysfunction. There are several manufacturers of external vacuum assist devices, most working on the same pump-applied vacuum system. I have chosen to describe the Erec-Aid vacuum assist device because its quality in design and manufacturing excellence is at a high level, because its makers' association with the renowned National Impotence Resource Center of the Osbon Foundation is a valuable resource of information and medical studies, and because I can speak about the ErecAid System from my own experience.

As a source of medical information on sexual erectile dysfunction, the Osbon Foundation in Augusta, Georgia, is unsurpassed. Geddings D. Osbon, Sr., was an inventive Georgia entrepreneur who suffered from erectile dysfunction. He refused to accept abstinence and did not want to give up the intimacy of sexual fulfillment with his dearly loved wife of thirty years. He worked tirelessly from 1961 to 1974, applying his particular combination of ingenuity, persistence, and faith to develop the Osbon vacuum assist device, which offers a practical and safe solution to impotence for millions of couples. Available by prescription since 1984, it is one of the most widely prescribed treatments for erectile dysfunction today.

The ErecAid vacuum assist device comes in its own fitted carrying case. The system is composed of the twelve-inch-long, clear cylindrical tube, a battery-powered pump, three-point tension rings, a squeeze tube of lubricant, and instructional materials. It is only available with a physician's prescription, which insures that you have consulted with your doctor concerning an erectile dysfunction problem.

Using the ErecAid device, I immediately became aware that some working experience would be necessary in order to successfully utilize the components to their fullest extent. For instance, you must carefully secure the pump to the opening at the top of the cylinder and insure that there are no air leaks at this juncture. If you loosely connect the pump, you will find you do not obtain a proper vacuum. It is also important to apply a liberal amount of lubricant to the bottom of the cylinder, so that a good juncture is made between the tube and the pubic area surrounding the penis. Again, if you do not have a good connection at this point, you will not easily obtain a vacuum.

Once you place the cylinder over the flaccid penis, with proper connection of the pump and lubricant applied, the pump is turned on. A negative pressure is created within the cylinder, causing blood to flow rapidly into the penis, as in a normal erection. If, using the palm of your left or right hand, a steady pressure is applied from the top of the pump downward, you will find it easier to obtain a vacuum. When a vacuum is felt on the penis, with some experience and technique, you can learn to adjust the vacuum control ring, thus allowing for additional vacuum or decreased vacuum as you adjust the ring or momentarily release the vacuum release valve. This enables you to continue the application of the vacuum as the penis becomes further engorged with blood and a good erection is achieved.

As the penis becomes fully erect, you may wish to slip onto the penis the three-point tension ring, a rubber ring with applied rubber "handles" that has been placed over the lower end of the cylinder. The tension ring is left on during intercourse. However, it should not be used longer than thirty minutes at a time.

Once you become adept at gaining a vacuum and obtaining an erection with the ErecAid device, you will find, as I did, that the device encourages blood flow into the penis and strengthens the vascular supply to the penis as you continue to use it. Do not become discouraged with your first attempts at using the ErecAid device. As you become more and more comfortable with it, you will find it a great asset to your total sexual health. I suggest learning to use the ErecAid device in private, and as you become more adept in its use, encouraging your partner to assist you. ErecAid maintains a twenty-four-hour telephone support system and clinical instruction program. One of the great advantages to this program is that it allows for the return to normal erections and normal potency, yet does not preclude the use of any of the other options. Clinical studies have suggested that there may be a great therapeutic benefit to increasing the number of penile blood vessels from repetitive use of external vacuum therapy. Some patients have done so well that they have regained normal function.

There are minimal side effects with external vacuum assist devices, including bruising, slight discomfort, and reddish pinpoint-sized dots appearing on the penis. Vacuum therapy should be used with caution in those diabetic patients with accompanying sickle-cell disease, leukemia, pelvic infections, or blood-clotting problems.

Self-Injection Therapy
If you have tried the vacuum assist device and you are still unable to gain and maintain an erection, there is a category of drugs with which you can inject yourself when an erection is desired. The best-studied and most effective drugs of this category are papaverine hydrochloride, phentolamine, and prostaglandin E1. Papaverine hydrochloride is a drug that is injected into the corpora cavernosa of the penis (see penile anatomy, this chapter). Injection therapy is relatively safe and erections are of good quality and appear natural. There is no need for any device to be worn during sexual intercourse, and partners need not know how the erection was produced. These drugs cause an engorgement of blood into the penis, causing an erection that typically lasts for one hour. The patient is taught to administer the injection himself, and the results have proved to be overwhelmingly positive. Your doctor must determine the correct dosage and teach the correct injection procedure. The only unwanted result of papaverine hydrochloride injections is that, in approximately 5–10 percent of users, there has been reported prolonged and painful erection, which may require an antidote injection or emergency treatment. Close follow-up by your doctor is required so that he or she may evaluate plaque formation, fibrosis, or scarring resulting from the injections. Your dosage level may require changes, the drug itself may have to be changed, or your doctor may prescribe several drug combinations to be injected. In-

jection therapy is not indicated in patients taking monoamine oxidase (MAO) inhibitors, so be sure to discuss all your medications with your physician. Use of penile injections is limited to two times per week, and side effects include infection, pain, bruises, fibrosis or scarring within the penis, priapism (prolonged painful erection), dizziness, elevated blood pressure, heart palpitations, or a flushed feeling.

Caverject is an FDA-approved form of injection therapy along with prostaglandin, and new medications are soon to be released.

Finally, a new system called MUSE, the new intraurethral delivery system of prostaglandin, has recently been approved for use by the FDA. Dr. Kenneth A. Goldberg says that MUSE works for approximately 40 percent of men and is certainly an option for consideration.

If you think you could benefit from these treatments, consultation with your doctor is the best way to begin. Your doctor may choose to send you to a specialist, such as a urologist who has experience in male sexual dysfunction, or he or she may choose to teach you the procedure. A urologist is a specially trained surgeon dealing in the diagnosis and treatment of the problems affecting the genitourinary tract, which includes the bladder, prostate, and genitals. Remember, only about one third of the urologists in the United States actively treat erectile dysfunction, so make sure the one you see does. In any case, study the possibilities and carefully evaluate this procedure.

As diabetic males, our sexuality is as important to us as for non-diabetic males, and it is paramount that we are able to enjoy our sexual life in as healthy and gratifying a manner as possible. Certainly, the diabetic condition has an effect on our sexuality and, as is the case in other areas of diabetic complications, it can produce some negative effects. We now know that maintaining our blood sugar levels within normal limits is vitally important to preventing complications of long-term diabetes. This applies equally well to the state of our sexual and reproductive organs because diabetes exerts its affect on our systems in total, not just in part. Poor diabetes management will cause adverse reactions to occur at all levels in our bodies.

21

How to Avoid Stress

Some years ago I visited the home of a good friend who is younger than I. We share a common interest in amateur radio and cars and also the fact that we are both diabetic and need to take twice-daily insulin injections.

We sat down at his kitchen table so that he could take his blood glucose reading and give himself an insulin injection. He brought his two vials of insulin and a syringe and alcohol pad to the table. He then made three successive trips from the table, one trip to get his glucose monitoring instrument, another to get his vial of strips, and—remembering his antihypertensive medication—a trip to the kitchen cabinet for this container of pills. Once he sat down again, he remembered his lancet and lancet-holding device, which meant another trip. By the time he was ready to take his blood sugar, he was a nervous wreck. This man was not only disorganized; he was working twice as hard to obtain a blood glucose reading and take his insulin injection as I do.

Instead of having separate places for all your diabetic equipment, store everything in a special medical bag; this will not only keep everything in one place, but will also make it more convenient to take along with you when you travel. When my friend followed this simple piece of advice, he immediately created a less stressful situation for himself. This man lived alone and there were several areas of his life that were totally disorganized. Diabetes must be placed in a part of your life that remains totally organized and disciplined.

Diabetes, in and of itself, can be the cause of a tremendous level of stress, frustration, and depression. We are living with an incurable disease that seems to have been here since the earliest recorded human history, and when all the items of the responsibility of diabetes are added up, it can be overwhelming.

For me, and for most successful diabetics, the most important component is keeping and maintaining an attitude of total positive thought and not dwelling on the negative aspects of this disease. Yes, I do live with total blindness every day. However, I do not get lost concentrating on how bad off I am. Instead, I work harder to achieve more and do what I can to improve my life and the lives of those around me.

At times it requires only a slight adjustment, as in the case of getting your diabetes medical supplies organized, and at other times it requires a total lifestyle adjustment, as I found out when I became blind. In both cases, mild and extreme, it is our determination to carry on with the most positive of thoughts that will enable us to survive.

Major psychosocial factors are involved with diabetes, whether the diabetic manages and copes well or is having an extremely difficult time accepting the disease. There is the requirement of learning a new lifestyle filled with new technical skills and jargon and the long-term determination to maintain this new life in the face of the progressive nature of diabetes. Stressful life situations, personality, family and social support, and environment are all important areas that contribute to the success or failure in handling the long-term nature of a chronic illness such as diabetes. Stress can be especially harmful for the diabetic, and if left unchecked, stress can lead to life-threatening consequences. I can speak from experience when it comes to stress. Since I verge on a Type A personality, there was a time in my life that just about anything at all could cause me an extreme amount of stress. Even things that I really enjoyed doing could stress me out. I believe now, after many years of reflection, that it was not the happy things in my life that caused my stress, but rather other areas that were so stressful that anything I did at all seemed to cause me stress.

My medical research work was extremely tedious and could be very frustrating; however, it was also a great challenge. The stress it created in my life was at times unmanageable. When I tried to do my favorite hobbies, such as Japanese gardening and bonsai-tree culturing, I would become stressed out. Working on my sports cars during the weekends caused me stress instead of joy. It finally dawned on me that I had to find the immediate cause of my stress and learn to deal with it in a manner suitable to the situation.

Once I identified the stressors, such as a sense of never being able to keep up with the medical literature in my field, never being able to publish enough scientific papers, seemingly endless clinical protocols to attend to, and other political situations in the office, I was able to place them in a rational level of priority and then deal with them in a logical manner. And I finally realized that I was not the only person in the world dealing with stress on a daily basis.

Obviously, overt stress is detrimental to the diabetic. Stress can cause your blood sugar to rise sharply, and due to the other hormones that can flare up during stress, you may not notice it until you test your blood sugar. My suggestion is that during times of great stress, take a few minutes, pull out your blood glucose monitor, and check your blood sugar. Not only will the result surprise you, but it will give you a few minutes to reflect upon whether the stress is necessary or unnecessary. Get up and walk around for a few minutes and take some deep breaths. This always seems to help when I am completely stressed out.

We do know that stress plays an influential role in the course of diabetes. Studies done in 1952 by Henkle and Wolfe and in 1974 by Grant and colleagues have found the following:

1. Stressful experiences can lead to changed behavior, including those of diet management, exercise, and insulin and blood glucose monitoring.
2. During stressful periods, metabolically influential agents, such as drugs and alcohol, may be used to quell upsets.
3. Altered emotional states may be accompanied by different hormone secretion patterns and thus influence diabetic blood glucose instability. Severe depression is often accompanied by shifts in the variation of the production of cortisol, a counterregulatory hormone. Other emotional upsets may influence other groups of hormones to cause changes in glucose and fat metabolism.

Clearly, there is a complex interaction between stress and the blood glucose level of the diabetic. The diabetic may experience wide variations in blood glucose values, either up or down, in response to emotionally upsetting conditions because different emotional states elicit the release of different combinations of stress-related hormones, which lead to a great variation in blood glucose values, both high and low. I know of several cases of diabetics who have experienced the loss or death of a loved one and had to be carefully watched by close friends and family to prevent them from falling into extreme states of low blood sugar.

The personality of an individual and the individual's ability to accept the chronic and progressive nature of diabetes vary greatly from person to person and may even vary greatly within the same diabetic from year to year. At some time during the life of most diabetics, partial or even total regimen abandonment can occur. Experts believe that the meticulous attention to the details required in dealing with diabetes over the long term can cause the individual to grow weary and give in to bad habits or neglect. Those diabetics who stay on track and try to maintain good control of their diabetes have fewer complications than those who fall victim to neglect. In many ways, the diabetic's control of his regimen is thought to be the key mechanism by which the individual's emotional state affects his metabolic control.

After a review of the literature concerning coping mechanisms and diabetes, I realized that one of my coping mechanisms during my earlier years with diabetes was rather common. My thinking was that I would rather maintain higher blood glucose levels than suffer an insulin reaction during periods of work that demanded my close attention to detail. This was a time before the common usage of self home blood glucose monitors; however, I could tell when my blood sugars were running high by the number of trips to the bathroom I made. There may be times when this particular coping mechanism is necessary, as when operating heavy machinery or driving an automobile. (Diabetes is not a legal excuse when an accident is caused by a diabetic driving under the influence of an insulin reaction.) When driving for long periods, I always kept a source of glucose, such as orange juice, candy bars, and hard candy, readily available.

Today, the medical management of diabetes is comprised of tight blood glucose control and intensified insulin therapy. We now know that this type of treatment greatly reduces the possibility of long-term complications such as diabetic retinopathy and nephropathy. Small portable blood glucose monitors make it easier to determine the blood glucose level. Keep in mind that trying to maintain normal blood glucose values will inevitably mean some hypoglycemic episodes. Therefore, you will have to learn how to manage this potentially serious problem. Decide how you will manage an insulin reaction at work. Make sure your coworkers and friends are aware of your diabetic condition and know how to assist you with orange juice or another source of glucose should you lapse into a serious insulin reaction.

The longer you have diabetes, the better you will be able to manage and cope with its many complexities. Make a promise to yourself that you will develop, from the outset, a mental framework of the most positive attitude and the best skills possible in self-managing your disease. Of utmost importance is your relationship with your doctor, as your doctor's objective approach will allow him or her to see items you have missed in managing your diabetes on a day-to-day basis.

22

Reflections on a Lifetime with Insulin-dependent Diabetes

As I look back over the last thirty-two years of living with insulin-dependent diabetes, I am struck by the level of progress that has been made to make the life of the diabetic better. I learned to use my first syringe and stainless steel needle at age fifteen. The glass syringe was a fine instrument, with a sintered, that is, ground glass, plunger, and it required a great deal of dexterity and technique to draw up two different types of insulin while keeping the plunger from sliding out of the barrel of the syringe body. The stainless steel needle had a very large bore, and if it were not kept sharp and free of barbs by sharpening it with wet metal oxide sandpaper, it could cause a great deal of pain.

The entire unit, syringe barrel, plunger, and needle, was stored in a glass jar filled with alcohol to which sterile gauze pads had been added and layered at the bottom of the jar. Once a week, the glass syringe assembly and needle had to be boiled thoroughly in order to sterilize them and to remove sticky insulin deposits. Every morning I fished my syringe out of the alcohol, dried it, and then attached the needle to the tip of the syringe. I then withdrew my proper insulin dose.

The diabetic of today uses disposable, microfine syringes, high-tech portable blood glucose monitors, and super pure human insulin preparations based on the internationally accepted one-hundred-unit scale. Diabetics can now control their blood sugar better than ever before because of the self home blood glucose monitor. With the release of the results of the Diabetes Control and Complications Trial (DCCT) in 1994, scientific evidence supports the fact that intensified insulin therapy and tight blood glucose control resembling the euglycemic or normal state means a decrease in such insidious diabetic complications as retinopathy, nephropathy, and neuropathy. Now not only do we have the doctors at the Joslin Diabetes Foundation and the American Diabetes Association telling us that tight blood glucose control prolongs our lives; we have a ten-year scientific study proving it.

So, why is diabetes still the number-one cause of new blindness in the United States? Why are more and more people becoming diabetic and tens of thousands dying from this disease every year? Unfortunately, we are still only managing this disease and not curing those who have it. The elusive enigma of the nature of this disease continues to baffle the world's scientists and medical researchers. However, if our medical technology continues at this accelerated rate, then the future holds the greatest potential for further unraveling the insidious nature of diabetes.

As I review my lifetime with diabetes, I believe that living with a positive attitude on a daily basis is the only way to go. During my two years of undiagnosed, uncontrolled diabetes I had deteriorated and wasted away; the combination of insulin injections and a healthy diet returned my strength and vigor. I went from failing my ninth grade strength and endurance tests in physical education to surfing big waves in the Hawaiian Islands just three years later. Without my loving family, insulin, healthy food, and a willingness to learn what seemed to be an insurmountable level of new lifestyle information, I would not have made it to the point of being able to write this book.

I have lived with total blindness now for twelve years. Diabetic retinopathy is a scourge to the life of any diabetic, and I found myself helpless in preventing its eventual outcome. Today the technology to save the eyesight of diabetics has dramatically improved. After my first two years of blindness, I was able to accept the condition at a better functioning level, and the rehabilitation training provided by state-run agencies for the blind is almost miraculous in turning the blind person's life around. Again, living life with a totally positive attitude is crucial, and the sooner you instill this type of philosophy in your life with diabetes, the better your life will become.

My life with blindness has evolved through a change in my consciousness level, my spirituality, and my intuitive and perceptual ability. It has led me to a world of close friendships that I may never have developed in my sighted life. I have had to learn adaptive methods in dealing with my daily insulin injections, taking my blood glucose readings, and participating in exercise and an active life. The most important aspect of all this is that it can be done, and I am living proof of this.

The new era of genetic engineering and hybrid cell technology may host untold benefits for the future of chronic metabolic diseases such as diabetes. As new ideas are planned, designed, and then parlayed into experimental protocol, the total effectiveness can be evaluated by using animal models. Clinical experiments can then be performed on human diabetic volunteer subjects, heralding a new treatment modality to improve the life of the diabetic patient.

Implantable cells with specific functions will take on more and more importance in the treatment of many human diseases, diabetes being one of the more notable. The race is well under way to develop an artificial pancreas for the diabetic. Many experimental designs have come and gone, most with some useful aspect, but usually accompanied by a major drawback that negates clinical application for its use within the diabetic population. A critical limiting factor has been developing an implantable sensor that allows continuous measurement of the circulating blood glucose and an effective feedback loop to tell the artificial pancreas when to release insulin and when to stop. It is indeed difficult to design a system that even comes close to mimicking the body's supreme method of endocrine control mechanisms.

Some of the latest techniques involved in the design of a biocompatible artificial pancreas include the transplantation of pancreatic islet cells with immuno-isolating membranes. As these cells are actually live transplanted pancreatic tissue, they must be encapsulated in order to be protected from attack by the body's own self-defense mechanisms. Specially designed, coated microcapsules, which are implanted in the peritoneum or abdominal cavity, or, alternatively, subcutaneously, have been found to perform quite well.

Over the past decade, several methods of microencapsulating pancreatic beta cells have shown great promise. Tiny microcapsules offer some distinct advantages over other implantable devices, one of the more important being delivery of the microcapsules into the peritoneum by use of a syringe. By simply injecting these microcapsules, if and when perfected, physiological glycemic control could take on a new definition. So far, the experimental protocols have been carried out on animals with good long-term results and without the use of immunosuppressive (antirejection) drugs. This is crucially important due to the wide range of deleterious side effects that long-term immunosuppressive drugs can cause.

I accept each day as a new challenge to live better, work and study more, play and exercise harder, enjoy the healthful benefits of a healthy diabetic diet, all the while living with the most positive mind-set of attitudinal healing. You can incorporate this vitally important attitude into your life with diabetes by working at it on a daily basis. If you do not see how this attitudinal healing can help you at this time, perhaps additional reading and study in this area may change your mind. The first step is just to be open to more of the possibilities than you ever thought of before.

Diabetes is a full-time challenge and will not ever give you a break, especially when you feel you need it the most. A special kind of stamina is required to live with this incurable disease for a lifetime, and special mental conditioning will certainly assist you. Your adherence to meticulous discipline and the necessary care your diabetes requires will also assist in getting you through the difficult times.

If this book has inspired you to learn more about diabetes and living a healthy lifestyle, then perhaps working in some area associated with diabetes, as a volunteer or a medical professional, would be something for you to consider. I have spent the last thirty years learning and studying about this disease, its etiology and elusive nature, and I do not plan on ever stopping. The study of diabetes is so fascinating and complex that any one area could create a lifetime of devoted study and work.

If you have ideas for the better health of the diabetic male, please write to me and share them with me, as this book can only begin to scratch the surface of the possibilities we may encounter. If you share my desire for better health and improved technology for the entire diabetic population, then join me in the enlightened pursuit for additional research into the molecular biology of diabetes, fair practice and attitudes toward diabetes in the workplace, and fair state and federal support of programs intended to better the life of the diabetic. Obviously, there is a tremendous amount of work that can be done. Perhaps you may be able to accomplish some great advancement toward the better understanding of this very ancient disease. Know from the beginning that my hopes and prayers for your success are with you.

Comments by Kenneth A. Goldberg, M.D., on Male Impotence and Diabetes

Erection problems are truly some of the most difficult but rewarding medical conditions I treat—not least of all because they involve two patients rather than one. When a man has an erection problem, his partner does too, and the result can be terribly destructive to a relationship. And just as they share the hardship, so must they cooperate on the solution. Understanding that it takes two to tango is the first step to solving a sexual problem—whatever it may be.

Although many if not most erection problems have a physical basis, particularly among diabetic men, every couple with an erection problem has an emotional problem as well. And the power of the mind when it comes to erections should never be discounted. Adrenaline can snuff out an erection in seconds, so a man who worries about his performance is a man who is unlikely to succeed. It takes support and love to get that tango going again.

Of course, as a diabetic man, you need to be particularly well informed about the physiological side of erectile dysfunction, because your condition does dramatically increase the risk. Diabetes, if not well controlled, threatens the very foundation of an erection: blood flow and nerves. An erection depends on clear arteries to fill the penis with blood and healthy penile tissues to prevent the blood from getting out. Likewise, diabetic neuropathy can affect the nerves that signal erection and those that control ejaculation and orgasm. And beyond the hard-penis problem, nerve damage can dull the sensitivity of the skin that provides sexual pleasure. As Dr. Juliano points out, prevention is the best treatment; if you control your diabetes, you can, in all likelihood, avoid such problems.

Fortunately, the news is good for all men who face erectile dysfunction. Medical science has advanced so much in the past ten years that I can say with confidence that any man can have an erection—and most without much difficulty. When I started medical practice in the late 1970s, we had only one solution to offer: the penile implant (or prosthesis). Those early devices caused more than a few problems, particularly in diabetic men. But today I'm happy to call the implant "the last resort." We have far better options to offer most men—and especially diabetics—and Dr. Juliano does a fine job of describing them in Chapter 20. As you read, however, remember that the best solution must suit both of you. If the time comes to choose one, make it a cooperative decision.

Finally, if you're a diabetic with an ongoing erection problem, don't give up on your sex life. Get help! I've treated men who hadn't had sex in years. Some of them successfully continue to use an erection aid. Others used an aid initially but now can get by on their own, just because they've gotten their confidence back. There's one thing they tell me they have in common, though, when they say, "Gee, Doc, I'd forgotten what I was missing!" Their partners say, "And how!"

Appendix B

The Symptoms
of Low Blood Sugar

Insulin reactions are undesirable at any time. They can even be dangerous, for example, while driving a car or in a remote setting where no one can see or assist you. *This is why, if you are at risk of having an insulin reaction, you should always carry a product such as Insta-Glucose with you.*

Mild Insulin Reaction:

You may suddenly feel shaky, nervous, very hungry, and sweaty.

Moderate Insulin Reaction:

If you do not notice or treat the mild reaction right away, it could progress to a moderate reaction with side effects such as headache, mood change, confusion, and a rapid heartbeat.

Severe Insulin Reaction:

Quick treatment of a mild or moderate reaction will help prevent a severe reaction. This stage usually requires assistance. You may lose consciousness and require an injection of glucagon or dextrose. Severe reactions do not happen very often when milder reactions are treated quickly.

Appendix C

Selected Newsletters
and Journals on Diabetes

Diabetes Quarterly Newsletter, a free information-packed newsletter.
The American Diabetes Association, Inc.
1660 Duke Street
Alexandria, VA 22314
Phone: (800) 232-3472

Diabetes Forecast, publication for diabetics.
The American Diabetes Association, Inc.
1660 Duke Street
Alexandria, VA 22314

Diabetes Interview, informative newspaper format with topics of interest to
those with diabetes.
3715 Balboa Street
San Francisco, CA 94121

The Diabetic Reader, an excellent newsletter dealing with current topics
related to diabetes by June Biermann and Barbara Toohey, authors of many
books about diabetes.
5623 Matilija Avenue
Van Nuys, CA 91401

Diabetes Self Management, Richard Rapaport, publisher; an excellent journal, published bimonthly, for those wishing to keep abreast of the latest
information concerning the self management of diabetes.
150 West 22nd Street
New York, NY 10011
Phone: (800) 234-0923

The Diabetic Traveler, an excellent newsletter for the diabetic who likes to travel.
P.O. Box 8223RW
Stamford, CT 06905

Voice of the Diabetic, Ed Bryant, editor; quarterly publication for visually impaired and blind diabetics prepared in print and audiocassette format by the Diabetic Division of the National Federation of the Blind.
811 Cherry Street, Suite 309
Columbia, MO 65201

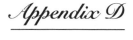

Other Resources

The American Diabetes Association, Inc.
Publishes *Diabetes Forecast* and other professional journals for the physician, medical researcher, and other health professionals.
1660 Duke Street
Alexandria, VA 22314

Bristol-Myers Squibb Pharmaceutical
Manufacturers of the ACE inhibitor captopril (Capoten) for the prolongation of the life of the diabetic kidney.
Bristol-Myers Squibb
U.S. Pharmaceutical
John Raia, Pharm.D.
777 Scutters Mill Road
Plainsboro, NJ 08543
Phone: (800) 321-1335

Health Care Products
Division of High Tech Pharmacal.
369 Bayview Avenue
Amityville, NY 11701
Phone: (800) 899-3116

ICN Pharmaceutical
Manufacturers of Insta Glucose, an excellent antihypoglycemic agent for treating insulin reactions.
Biomedical Division
3300 Hyland Avenue
Costa Mesa, CA 92626
Phone: (800) 431-1237

Eli Lilly and Company
World's largest manufacturer of insulin.
Lilly Corporate Center
Indianapolis, IN 46285

The Male Health Institute
Kenneth A. Goldberg, M.D.
Director
400 West LBJ Freeway, Suite 360
Dallas, TX 75063
Phone: (800) 422-6253

Medic Alert Foundation
P.O. Box 1009
Turlock, CA 95381
Phone: (800) 344-3226

Medical Hair Restoration
Matt Leavit, M.D.
Director
P.O. Box 940699
Maitland, FL 32794

National Impotence Resource Center
The Osbon Foundation
1246 Jones Street
PO Box 1593
Augusta, GA 30903-1593
Phone: (800) 433-4215

NordicTrack
104 Peavey Road
Chasca, MN 55318
Phone: (800) 328-5888

Nutrition Headquarters, Inc.
Manufacturers of Vitamins for Hair Care.
One Nutrition Plaza
Carbondale, IL 62901
Phone: (800) 851-3551

Progressive Research Lab
9219 Katy Freeway, Suite 162
Houston, TX 77024
Phone: (800) 877-0966

Raintree Group, Inc.
Specializes in herbal products from the Amazon rain forest, with over sixty
rain-forest plants currently under research, many of which are beneficial to
the diabetic.
1601 West Koenig Lane
Austin, TX 78756
Phone: (512) 467-6130 or (800) 780-5902

Silva International
Jose Silva
P.O. Box 2249
1407 Calle del Norte
Laredo, TX 78044
Emax, Inc.
Distributors of diabetic care products for skin, feet, and joints formulated
with oil from the Australian emu.
Phone: 1-888-485-7844 or (409) 968-4903

O. Carl Simonton, M.D., Cancer Counseling and Research Center
Tapes and Literature
PO Box 623
Bridgeport, TX 76246
Phone: (800) 338-2360
Patient Care
PO Box 890
Pacific Palisades, CA 90272
Phone: (800) 459-3424

Texas College of Traditional Chinese Medicine
Dr. Jeff Tsing
4045 Manchaca Road
Austin, TX 78704
Phone: (512) 444-8082

Wound Care Center of North Texas
Ron Scott, M.D.
8210 Walnut Hill Lane, Suite 718
Dallas, TX 75231
Phone: (214) 345-4114

Appendix E

Resource Guide to
Aids and Appliances

Published by the Diabetes Action Network
of the National Federation of the Blind

This resource list was developed by my friend and fellow blind diabetic, Ed Bryant, president of the Diabetes Action Network headquartered in Bethesda, Maryland.

Ed is editor of the *Voice of the Diabetic* (see page 178) and has taken the lead in convincing the Federal Food and Drug Administration and Eli Lilly, the world's leader in insulin manufacturing, to modify the vials of different insulins so that blind and visually impaired diabetics may differentiate one insulin type from another. Ed has successfully convinced insulin manufacturers that input from the visually impaired diabetic community is important.

General and Miscellaneous

Becton Dickenson Consumer Products, One Becton Drive, Franklin Lakes, NJ 07417-1883; phone: (800) 237-4554.

B-D Home Sharps Container: 1.5-quart leak-proof container holds seventy to one hundred used syringes for safe disposal.

B-D Safe-Clip: Safely removes and stores used syringe needles prior to disposal.

Boehringer Mannheim Corporation, 9115 Hague Road, Indianapolis, IN 46250-0100; phone: (800) 428-5074; fax: (317) 576-3070.

Accu-Drop Blood Sample Device: Uses ChemStrip BG test strips. May aid placement of blood on strip.

Carolyn's Catalog, P.O. Box 14577, Bradenton, FL 34280-4577; phone: (800) 648-2266. Adaptive equipment distributor; free catalog (standard print only).

Digital Blood Pressure Meter: Easy-to-read large LCD readout; automatic power-off function.

Jordan Medical Enterprises, 12555 Garden Grove Boulevard, Suite 507, Garden Grove, CA 92643; phone: (800) 541-1193.

Count-A-Dose Insulin Measuring Device: Gauge calibrated for use with U-100 vials and B-D $1/2$-cc (low dose) syringes only. By turning a thumb-wheel, clicks are heard and felt for each one-unit increment measured; holds one or two vials of insulin for mixing; needle penetrates vial stopper automatically. Print and excellent cassette instruction provided.

LS & S Group, P.O. Box 673, Northbrook, IL 60065; phone: (800) 468-4789. Adaptive equipment distributor; catalog free in print.

Thermakit Insulin Container: Insulated container reduces agitation, protects against temperature fluctuations. Holds two insulin vials and two syringes (any brand).

Pill-Alert: Interval timer/alarm pillbox can be set to beep every four to sixteen hours; LCD display; battery included.

Med-Safe Systems, Inc., 4665 North Avenue, Oceanside, CA 92056-3590; phone: (800) 268-2001.

Insulin Syringe and Lancet Disposal System: Resembles a tissue box, holds up to one hundred used syringes. Starter kit, with decorative cover and three refills. Refills sold separately in sets of three.

Medicool, Inc., 23761 Madison Street, Torrence, CA 90505; phone: (800) 433-2469; in CA call: (800) 654-1565.

Insulin Protector Case: A specially designed case that will keep insulin cool for up to sixteen hours while traveling; also holds syringes, swabs, or test strips.

Meditec, Inc., 3322 S. Oneida Way, Denver, CO 80224; phone: (303) 758-6978.

Holdease: Needle guide and syringe/vial holder; holds syringe and vial together for filling operation, use with Insulgage (below) for nonsighted filling. Works with all U-100 syringes.

Insulgage: Flat plastic insulin gauge slips onto B-D or Monoject 1-cc or $1/2$-cc syringe, allows tactile draw-up of preset dose. Many sizes available, one per Insulgage. Available in several formats including Braille with raised numbers.

Novo Nordisk Pharmaceuticals Inc., 100 Overlook Center, Suite 200, Princeton, NJ 08540; phone: (800) 727-6500. Novo Nordisk states: "None of our devices are recommended for use by blind or visually impaired persons without sighted aid." Both products use PenNeedle disposable needles (sold separately).

Novolin Pen Insulin Delivery System: Made of durable plastic; uses Novolin cartridges, regular, NPH, or 70/30 human insulin. Measures insulin in even increments from two to thirty-six units. A click is heard for each two units of insulin drawn. Difficulties have been reported with the reliability of the click for measuring purposes.

Novolin Prefilled: Disposable dial-a-dose syringe holds 150 units of R, 70/30, or N human insulin; measures two to fifty-eight units in two-unit increments.

Owen Mumford, Inc., 849 Pickens Industrial Drive, Suite 12, Marietta, GA 30062; phone: (800) 421-6936.

Autopen Insulin Delivery System: Made in England; uses Novolin insulin cartridges and needles; two models, one that clicks for each unit drawn, from one to sixteen units, and the other that clicks at each two-unit increment, with a range of two to thirty-two units.

Palco Labs, Inc., 8030 Soquel Avenue, #104, Santa Cruz, CA 95062; phone: (800) 346-4488; fax: (408) 476-1114.

Insul-Tote: All-weather insulated tote transports insulin, meter, and strips. Four models.

Load-Matic: Tactile insulin measuring device, accepts B-D 100 unit syringe; aligns needle with vial stopper; two separate controls (one for single unit and the other for ten-unit increments); tactile prompt to confirm dose setting. Cassette instructions. Individuals with neuropathy may have difficulty with the one-unit scale, and it is possible to unintentionally "short-stroke" the ten-unit loading lever and draw an incomplete dose.

Science Products, Box 888, Southeastern, PA 19399; phone: (800) 888-7400. Free print catalog.

Good Health Combo: This three-unit talking health kit monitors blood pressure and takes temperature. Same voice box works with both blood pressure monitor and thermometer. Both measuring units present readings in spoken and extralarge (about two inches high) LCD display. The blood pressure monitor gives date, time, systolic/diastolic, and pulse readings; comes with a printer and rechargeable battery; stores seven readings; weighs twenty-nine ounces; the temperature monitor weighs five ounces. Purchased separately, thermometer comes with a cable and is voice-ready; has large LCD display but has no voice. Blood pressure monitor can also be purchased separately and works as described above.

Automatic Insulin Injection Systems

Health-Mor Personal Care Corp., 185 E. North Street, Bradley, IL 60915; phone: (800) 991-4464.

AdvantaJet Needle-Free Injection System: Automatic jet-stream injection system; tactile detents for each unit drawn. Cost includes training, twenty-four-hour help line, free loaner.

Jordan Medical Enterprises, 12555 Garden Grove Boulevard, Suite 507, Garden Grove, CA 92643; phone: (800) 541-1193.

Instaject: Shatterproof combination insulin injector/blood lancet device; fits all sizes/brands of insulin syringes (except Monoject) without adapters. Can be adjusted for depth of needle penetration; fits in palm of hand; fits many lancets.

Medi-Ject, 1840 Berkshire Lane, Minneapolis, MN 55441; phone: (800) 328-3074.

Medi-Jector (MJ6): Needle-free injector, measures in one-half–unit increments; tactile and visual cues. With practice, should be suitable for independent use by the blind. Two versions: adult and pediatric.

Owen Mumford, Inc., 849 Pickens Industrial Drive, Suite 12, Marietta, GA 30062; phone: (800) 421-6936.

Autoject 2: An update of the Autojector. Two models (fixed-needle or disposable-needle syringes); injects the needle at a prescribed depth; incorporates safety lock. Uses all syringe types.

Palco Labs, Inc., 8030 Soquel Avenue, Santa Cruz, CA 95062; phone: (800) 346-4488; fax: (408) 476-1114.

Inject-Ease: Can be used with most low-dosage syringes; with B-D syringes, cap can be left on needle while loading device. Five-year warranty.

Sherwood Medical, Consumer Department, 1831 Olive Street, St. Louis, MO 63103; phone: (314) 621-7788. Free information pamphlet available.

Monoject Injectomatic: Requires use of Monoject syringes. When pressed against injection site, needle is injected. Two sizes: 1 cc (hundred-unit syringes) or $^{1}/_{2}$ cc (fifty-unit syringes).

Vitajet Corporation, 27075 Cabot Road, #102, Laguna Hills, CA 92653; phone: (714) 582-0713.

Vitajet: Needle-free insulin injector; delivers from two to fifty units; adjustable jet pressure; some capacity for mixing insulins; raised dosage scale and some tactile cues facilitate low-vision administration. Three-year warranty.

Blood Glucose Monitoring Systems

GLUCOMETERS WITH VOICE EMULATION
Home Diagnostics, Inc., 2300 NW 55th Court, Suite 110, Ft. Lauderdale, FL 33309; phone: (800) 342-7226; fax: (908) 542-6754.

LifeScan, Inc., 1051 S. Milpitas Boulevard, Milpitas, CA 05035; phone: (800) 227-8862.

One Touch Profile: Successor to the One Touch II; same strips, operating instructions, and accuracy; features vastly expanded internal memory and functions. Offered by many suppliers.

NONTALKING GLUCOMETERS

Bayer Corporation, Diagnostics Division, Elkhart, IN 46515; phone: (800) 348-8100.

Glucometer Elite: Large display; no timing, wiping, or cleaning.

LifeScan, Inc., 1051 S. Milpitas Boulevard, Milpitas, CA 05035; phone: (800) 227-8862.

One Touch Basic: Simple and reliable procedures; large LCD readout; easy to clean.

MediSense, Inc., 266 Second Avenue, Waltham, MA 02154; phone: (800) 527-3339.

Precision QID: Large LCD readout; simplified operating drill; uses both MediSense strips and Precision QID Microflo strips, the latter allowing strip to be touched and machine to be moved while testing.

Insulin Pumps

Disetronic Medical Systems, Inc., 5201 E. River Road, Suite 312, Minneapolis, MN 55421-1014; phone: (800) 688-4578.

H-Tron V Insulin Pump: Insulin delivery system mimics natural pancreas; requires training to use; suitable for use by highly motivated diabetics; user can program two types of insulin delivery methods; "basal" rate and "bolus" dose; weighs less than three and a half ounces, including batteries; acoustic signals for stop, run, bolus, basal rate, reduction, warnings, and alarms. Various information displays on LCD readout; uses two three-volt silver oxide batteries.

Mini Med, 12744 San Fernando Road, Sylmar, CA 91342; phone: (800) 440-7867

Mini Med 507 Insulin Pump: This new version is the most current model, which packages control, freedom, and safety in a sophisticated new design. It incorporates flexibility and reliability for the precise control of insulin delivery to lessen diabetic complications.

Large Distributors of Diabetes Equipment and/or Supplies

These distributors have retail sales outlets in their respective locations. All offer free catalogs.

Diabetes Self-Care (formerly Sugar-Free Center), 3601 Thirlane Road, N.W., Suite 4, Roanoke, VA 24019; phone: (800) 258-9559. Full line of diabetes equipment and pharmaceuticals; phone and in-home training; direct billing of insurance claims.

Diabetes Supplies, 6505 Rockside Road, Suite 325, Independence, OH 44131; phone: (800) 622-5587. Sales tax on applicable items in Ohio. No third-party insurance carriers accepted.

Home Service Medical, Inc., P.O. Box 59024, Minneapolis, MN 55459-9685; phone: (800) 876-6540. Nominal handling charge on small orders; no charge on larger orders. Sales tax charged in Minnesota on insulin and syringes. Third-party insurance carriers accepted on a qualified basis. Medicare accepted nationally, Medicaid in Minnesota only.

Liberty Medical Supply, 3595 S.W. Corporate Parkway, Palm City, FL 34990; phone: (800) 762-8026. More than one hundred different items stocked. Medicare or private insurance accepted. Most orders shipped free.

St. Louis Medical Supply, 10821 Manchester Road, Kirkwood, MO 63122; phone: (800) 950-6020; in MO call: (314) 821-7355; fax: (314) 821-5102. Small handling charge for all orders. Sales tax on all Missouri orders except insulin.

Stadtlanders, 600 Penn Center Boulevard, Pittsburgh, PA 15235-5810; phone: (800) 238-7828. Stadtlanders pharmacy program offers medication, delivery, and insurance billing services. Diabetics, organ transplant recipients, and others are provided with free express medication delivery anywhere in the U.S.

Selected Readings

Chapter 1: Gaining a Perspective on Diabetes
McGrew, Roderick E. *Encyclopedia of Medical History*. New York: McGraw-Hill, 1985, p. 93.
Walton, John, Paul Beeson, and Ronald Bodley Scott, eds. *The Oxford Companion to Medicine*. New York: Oxford University Press, 1986, vol. 1, p. 308.

Chapter 2: Insulin
Ellenberg, Max, and Harold Rifkin, eds. *Diabetes Mellitus: Theory and Practice*. 3rd ed. Paramus, New Jersey: Prentice Hall, 1988, pp. 777–90.

Chapter 3: Oral Antidiabetic Medications
Oral Diabetes Medication Pills to Treat Type II Diabetes. Alexandria, Virginia: American Diabetes Association, 1996.

Chapter 5: Clinical Blood Tests
Bunn, H. F., A. Gab, and P. M. Gallup. "The Non-Enzymatic Glycosylation of Hemoglobin and the Glycosylation of Hemoglobin: Relevance to Diabetes Mellitus." *Science* 200 (1978): 21.
Goldstein, D. E., R. R. Little, H. Weidmeir, et al. "Glycated Hemoglobin: Methodologies and Clinical Applications." *Clinical Chemistry* 32 (1986): B-64.
Moore, W. Tad, and Richard Eastman. *Diagnostic Endocrinology*. Philadelphia: B. C. Decker, 1990.

Chapter 8: Long-term Complications to the Diabetic Eye
April, Earnest W. *Anatomy*. 2nd ed. National Medical Series for Independent Study. Media, Pennsylvania: John Wiley & Sons, Harwal Publishing, John Wiley & Sons, 1990, pp. 457–82.
Garcia, Charles A., and Richard S. Ruiz. "Occular Complications of Diabetes." *Ciba Geigy Clinical Symposia* 44, no. 1 (1992).

Gray, Henry. *Gray's Anatomy*. 36th ed. Edited by Peter L. Williams and Roger Warwick. Philadelphia: W. B. Saunders, 1980, pp. 1150–89.

Chapter 9: Long-term Complications to the Diabetic Kidney
April, Earnest W. *Anatomy*. 2nd ed. National Medical Series for Independent Study. Media, Pennsylvania: John Wiley & Sons, Harwal Publishing, John Wiley & Sons, 1990, pp. 210–41.
National Diabetes Data Group. "Diabetes in America: Diabetes Data Compiled for 1984." Rockville, Maryland: NIH Publication Number 85 1468, pp. 269–99. August 1985.
Whelton, Paul K. "Preventing End Stage Renal Disease." *Scientific American Science and Medicine* (November–December 1994): 8.

Chapter 10: Long-term Complications to the Diabetic Vascular and Nervous Systems
Ellenberg, Max, and Harold Rifkin, eds. *Diabetes Mellitus: Theory and Practice*. 3rd ed. Paramus, New Jersey: Prentice Hall, 1988, pp. 777–90.

Chapter 11: Implications of Hypertension for the Diabetic
Chercliff, D. *Some Characteristics Related to Incidence of Coronary Disease and Death, Framingham Study Eighteen-Year Follow-up*. Washington, D.C.: U.S. Government Printing Office, 1974, p. 30.
Chrysant, Steven G. "The Losinopril-Hydrochlorothiazide Group: Low Dose Combination Therapy." *Archives of Internal Medicine* 154 (April 11, 1994): 737–743.
Crawl, F. D., and W. C. Roberts. *American Journal of Medicine* 64 (1978): 221.
Croog, Sidney, et al. "The Quality of Life Study." *New England Journal of Medicine* 314 (June 26, 1986): 1657–64.
Dzau, V., G. H. Gibbons, and R. E. Pratt. "Local Renin-Angiotensin System." *Hypertension*, 16, supp. II (1991): 100–105.
Endre, T., et al. "Insulin Resistance in Normotensive Relatives of Hypertensives." *Journal of Hypertension*, 12 (January 1994): 81–88.
Johnston, Colin I. "Tissue Angiotensin Converting Enzyme in Cardiac and Vascular Hypertrophy Repair and Remodeling." *Hypertension* 23 (February 1994): 258–268.
Lewis, E. J., et al. "Captopril and Diabetic Nephropathy." *New England Journal of Medicine* 329 (November 11, 1993): 1456–1462.
Opie, Lionel H. *Angiotensin Converting Enzyme Inhibitors: Scientific Basis for Clinical Use*. New York: Wiley Publishing, 1992.
Opie, Lionel H. "ACE Inhibitors: Almost Too Good to be True." *Scientific American Science and Medicine* (March–April 1995): 14–24.
Satoro, D. et al. "ACE Inhibition, Glucose Tolerance, and Insulin Sensitivity." *Hypertension* 20 (August 1992): 181–91.

Chapter 12: Taking a Positive Approach
Ornstein, Robert, and Charles Swencionis. *The Healing Brain: A Scientific Reader.* New York: Guilford Press, 1990.

Chapter 13: Exercise Physiology and Diabetes
Ellenberg, Max, and Harold Rifkin. *Diabetes Mellitus: Theory and Practice.* 3rd ed. Paramus, New Jersey: Prentice Hall, 1988, pp. 567–72.
NordicTrack Corporation. "Position Paper on Cross Country Skiing." Available from NordicTrack Corporation, 104 Peavey Road, Chaska, Minnesota, 1994.
Rollo, J. "Cases of Diabetes Mellitus with the Results of the Trials of Certain Acids and Other Substances." In *Cures of Louis Veneria*, 2nd ed., London, 1798.

Chapter 14: Acupunture and Diabetes
Omura, Yoshiaki. *Acupuncture Medicine: Its Historical and Clinical Background.* Tokyo: Japan Publications, 1982.
Omura, Y. "Acupuncture and Electro-therapeutics Research." *The International Journal* 1 (1975): 3–44.
Warren, Frank Z. and Masaru Toguchi. *The Complete Guide to Acupuncture and Acupressure.* 2 vols. in 1. Reprint, New York: Random House Value Publishing, 1991.

Chapter 15: The Diabetic Diet
Agriculture Handbook: Composition of Foods, Raw, Processed and Prepared. Washington, D.C.: U.S. Government Printing Office, 1994.
Anderson, James W. *Diabetes: A Practical New Guide to Healthy Living.* New York: Warner Books, 1983.
Juliano, Joseph and Dianne Young. *The Diabetic's Innovative Cookbook.* New York: Henry Holt, 1994.
Logan, James S. "Report on Soluble Fiber to the NANCI Corporation." Lecture. Tulsa, Oklahoma., 1991.
"Nutritional Recommendations and Principles for Individuals with Diabetes Mellitus." *Diabetes Care* 14, Supp. 2 (March 1991).
"Oat Bran: Some Like It Hot." *University of California Wellness Letter.* 1990.
Simms, Dorothea F. *Diabetes: Guide to Health and Freedom.* St. Louis, Missouri: C. V. Mosby, p. 27.
Wedman, Betty. *American Diabetes Association Holiday Cookbook.* New York: American Diabetes Association, 1986, Chap. 1.

Chapter 16: Vitamins
Bauernfeind, J. C. *The Safe Use of Vitamin A.* Washington, D.C.: ILSI Press, 1980.

Briggs, M. H., ed. *Recent Vitamin Research.* Boca Raton, Florida: CRC Press, Franklin, 1984.

Carpenter, Kenneth J. *The History of Scurvy and Vitamin C.* New York: Cambridge University Press, 1986.

Deigen, Jan B. *Vitamins and Memory: Niacin and Vitamin B6 in Age Related Cognitive Decline.* IBB, 1993.

Giller, Robert M. *Natural Prescriptions: Dr. Giller's Natural Treatments and Vitamin Therapies for More Than One Hundred Common Ailments.* New York: Ballantine, 1985.

Hayaishi, Osamu. *Clinical and Nutritional Aspects of Vitamin E.* New York: Elsevier, 1987.

Jacobs, Maryce M. *Vitamins and Minerals in the Treatment and Prevention of Cancer.* Boca Raton, Florida: CRC Press, 1991.

Lee, William. *Raw Fruit and Vegetable Juices and Drinks.* New Canaan, Connecticut: Keats, 1982.

Lonsdale, Derrick. *A Nutritionist's Guide to the Clinical Use of Vitamin B1.* Tacoma, Washington: Life Science Press, 1988.

Marshall, Charles W. *Vitamins and Minerals: Help or Harm.* Philadelphia: Lippincott, 1985.

Mindell, Earl. *Earl Mindell's Vitamin Bible.* New York: Warner Books, 1991.

Richards, Evelleen. *Vitamin C and Cancer: Medicine or Politics.* New York: St. Martin's Press, 1991.

Rosenbaum, Michael E. *Super Fitness Beyond Vitamins.* New York: NAL-Dutton, 1989.

Sauberlich, Howerde E. *Beyond Efficiency: New Views on the Function and Health Effects of Vitamins.* New York: New York Academy of Science, 1992.

Smith, L. H., ed. *Clinical Guide to the Use of Vitamin C.* Tacoma, Washington: Life Science Press, 1988.

Chapter 18: Dental Hygiene

Ellenberg, Max, and Harold Rifkin. *Diabetes Mellitus: Theory and Practice.* 3rd ed. Paramus, New Jersey: Prentice Hall, 1988, pp. 895–901.

Chapter 20: Erectile Dysfunction in the Diabetic Male

Danov, Dudley. *Super Potency.* New York: Time Warner, 1993.

Delliveau, Fred, and Lynn Richter. *Understanding Human Sexual Inadequacy.* New York: Bantam, 1970.

The Diagram Group. *Man's Body: An Owner's Manual.* New York: Paddington Press, Two Continent Publishing Group, 1976.

Ferrell, Warren. *The Myth of Male Power.* New York: Simon and Schuster, 1993.

Goldstein, Irwin, and Larry Rothstein. *The Potent Male*. Los Angeles: Price, Stern, Sloan, 1990.

Kaplan, Helen Singer. *Overcoming Premature Ejaculation*. New York: Brunner/Mazel, 1989.

Kaplan, Helen. *The Illustrated Manual of Sex Therapy*. New York: Quadrangle-New York Times, 1975.

Kelly, Gary F. *Good Sex: A Healthy Man's Guide to Sexual Fulfillment*. Orlando, Florida: Harcourt Brace Jovanovich, 1979.

Kolodny, Robert C., William H. Masters, and Virginia E. Johnson. *Textbook of Sexual Medicine*. Boston, Massachusetts: Little, Brown, 1979.

Lafavorae, Markel. *Men's Health Adviser*. Emmaus, Pennsylvania: Rodale Press, 1992.

Masters, William H., Virginia E. Johnson, and Robert C. Kolodny. *Human Sexuality*. 3rd ed. Boston, Massachusetts: Little, Brown, 1988, pp. 71–79, 80–91, 500–50.

Osbon Foundation. *Male Impotence: A Treatment Guide*. Atlanta, Georgia: Osbon Foundation, 1993.

Chapter 21: How to Avoid Stress

Cochran, H., A. Marble, and J. Galloway. "Factors in the survival of patients with insulin-requiring diabetes for 50 years." *Diabetes Care 2*, no. 4 (1979): 363–68.

Grant, I., G. C. Kyle, et al. "Recent life events and diabetes in adults." *Psychosomatic Medicine 36*, no. 2 (1974): 121–28.

Bibliography

Ahuja, M. M. *Practice of Diabetes Mellitus.* Vikas, India: Vikas Press.

American Dietetic Association Family Cookbook. Vols. I–II. New York: American Diabetes Association, 1986.

Arasham, Gary, and Earnest Lowe. *Diabetes: A Guide to Living Well.* Minnetonka, MN: DCI Publishing, 1988.

Berg, Krif E. *The Diabetics Guide to Health and Fitness.* Champaign, IL: Human Kinetics Publishing, 1986.

Bernstein, Richard K. *Food for Diabetes: The Glucograph Method for Normalizing Blood Sugars.* Los Angeles, CA: Jeremy P. Tarcher, 1984.

Bierman, June, and Barbara Toohey. *The Diabetics Total Health Book.* Los Angeles, CA: Jeremy P. Tarcher, 1988.

Binefield, Harriet, and Effram Corngold. *Between Heaven and Earth: A Guide to Chinese Medicine.* New York: Ballantine Books, 1992.

Blanchard, Pat. *Basic Menus and Recipes for Diabetics.* Creole Publishing, 1989.

Boucher, B. J., and Ian S. Raw. *Diabetes Mellitus: Laboratory Tests and Self Monitoring.* England: Wolfe Medical Books, 1988.

Bouloux, Pierre, and Leslie H. Rees. *Diagnostic Tests in Endocrinology and Diabetes, Diagnostic Test Survey.* Vol. 4. Chapman and Hall Publishing, 1993.

Bowens, Angela. *The Diabetic Gourmet.* New York: Harper & Row, 1981.

Brisco, Paula. *Diabetes: Questions You Have, Answers You Need.* Allentown, PA: Peoples Med Association Publishing, 1993.

Budd, Martin. *Diets to Help Diabetics.* London, England: Thorsons Sterling, 1988.

Cavaiani, Mabel. *The High Fiber Cookbook for Diabetics.* New York: Putnam Publishing Group, 1987.

Caditz, Judith. *Diabetes, Visual Impairment and Group Support: A Guide Book.* Center for the Partially Sighted, 1989.

Covelli, Pasquale, and Melvin Wiedman. *Diabetes: Current Research and Future Direction and Management and Cure.* Jefferson, NC: MacFarland and Company, 1988.

Creutzfeldt, W. *Acarbose for the Treatment of Diabetes Mellitus.* New York: Springer-Verlag, 1988.

Cooper, Kenneth H. *Controlling Cholesterol.* New York: Bantam Books, 1988.

DCCT Research Group, "The Effect of Intensive Treatment of Diabetes ..." *New England Journal of Medicine* 329 (1993) 977–86. Massachusetts Medical Society.

Developing Programs to Control and Prevent Diabetes: Analysis of the Problem. Austin, TX: LBJ School of Public Affairs, 1982.

Draznin, Boris, ed. *Molecular and Cellular Biology of Diabetes Mellitus.* Vols. 1–3. 1989.

Dolinar, Richard, and Betty P. Brackinridge. *Diabetes 101, a Pure and Simple Guide for People Who Use Insulin.* 2nd ed. Minnetonka, MN: Chronimed Press, 1993.

Ellis, Pat. *Cleveland Clinic Foundation Creative Cooking for Renal Diabetic Diets.* Cleveland: Cleveland Clinic Foundation and the Department of Nutrition Staff, Senay Publishers, 1987.

Finsand, Mary J. *Diabetic Cakes, Pies and Other Scrumptious Desserts.* New York: Sterling Press, 1988.

Franz, Marion. *Diabetes and Alcohol.* Minnetonka, MN: DCI Publishing, 1983.

Franz, Marion. *Diabetes and Exercise: A Complete Exercise Guide for People With Diabetes or Other Chronic Health Problems.* Minnetonka, MN: DCI Publishing, 1990.

Garell, Dale C., and Soloman H. Snyder. *Diabetes.* New York: Chelsea House Publishing, 1989.

Gordon, Neil F. *Diabetes: Your Complete Exercise Guide.* Champaign, IL: Human Kinetics Press, 1993.

Goren, Joseph H., ed. *Insulin Action in Diabetes.* New York: Raven Press, 1988.

Johnson, John. *Disorders of Sexual Potency in the Male.* Elmsford, NY: Pergammon Press, 1968.

Juliano, Joseph. *When Diabetes Complicates Your Life.* Minneapolis, MN: Chronimed DCI Publishing, 1993.

Juliano, Joseph, and Dianne Young. *The Diabetic's Innovative Cookbook.* New York: Henry Holt, 1994.

Julty, Sam. *Male Sexual Performance.* New York: Grossett and Dunlap, 1975.

Kozak, George P. *Management of Diabetic Foot Problems.* Philadelphia, PA: Saunders Publishing, 1984.

Laron, Z., and M. Karp. "Pre-Diabetes, Are We Ready to Intervene." *Pediatric and Adolescent Endocrinology* 23 (1993).

Levy, Linda, and Francine Grabowski. *Low Fat Living for Real People.* New York: Lake Isle Press, 1994.

Lodowick, Peter A. *A Diabetic Doctor Looks at Diabetes, His and Yours.* Cambridge, MA: R.M.I. Corporation, 1982.

Mark, Vernon, and Jeffrey Piedmark. *Brain Power: A Neurosurgeon's Complete Program to Maintain and Enhance Brain Fitness Throughout Your Life.* Boston, MA: Houghton Miflin, 1989.

Meyer, John K., Chester W. Schmidt, and Thomas N. Wise, eds. *Clinical Management of Sexual Disorders.* 2nd ed. Baltimore, MD: Williams and Wilkins, 1983.

Mimura, T. *Diabetes Mellitus in East Asia: Proceedings of the First China-Japan Symposium on Diabetes Mellitus.* Bejing, China, May 1988.

Moller, David, ed. *Insulin Resistance.* New York: John Wiley, 1993.

Nutrition of the Diabetic Child: Proceedings of the Fourth Beilinson Symposium, May 21–24, 1978. S. Karger Publisher, 1980.

Ornish, Dean. *Eat More, Weigh Less.* New York: HarperCollins, 1993.

Ornstein, Robert, and Charles Swencionis. *The Healing Brain: A Scientific Reader.* New York: Guilford Press, 1990.

Skillman, Thomas G., and Manuel Tzagournis. *Diabetes Mellitus*. Kalamazoo, MI: The Upjohn Company, 1983.

Simonton, O. Carl and James Creighton. *Getting Well Again*. Los Angeles: Jeremey Torher, 1978.

Simonton, O. Carl, and Reed M. Hanson. *The Healing Journey*. New York: Bantam Books, 1992.

Slyvjerg, Allan, et al. *Growth Hormone: An Insulin-Like Growth Factor I in Human and Experimental Diabetes*. New York: John Wiley, 1993.

Sobel, David. *The Healing Brain: Breakthrough Medical Discoveries About How the Brain Health Manages*. New York: Simon and Schuster, 1988.

Wetcher, Kenneth, Art Barker, and F. Rex McArtry. *Save the Males: Why Men Are Mistreated, Misdiagnosed, and Misunderstood*. Washington, DC: P.I.A. Press, 1991.

Zilbergel, Bernie. *The New Male Sexuality*. Boston, MA: Little, Brown, 1993.

*Supplemental Bibliography on Hypertension
from John Raia, Pharm.D.,
Bristol-Myers Squibb Pharmaceutical*

Anderson, S. and B. M. Brenner. "Therapeutic implications of converting enzyme inhibitors in renal disease." *American Journal of Kidney Disease* 1987; 10 (Suppl 1): 81–87.

Bauer, J. H., G. P. Reams, J. Hewett, D. Klachko, A. Lau, C. Messina, et al. "A randomized, double-blind, placebo-controlled trial to evaluate the effect of enalapril in patients with clinical diabetic nephropathy." *American Journal of Kidney Disease* 1992; 20: 443–457.

Bjorck, S., G. Nyberg, H. Mulec, et al. "Beneficial effects of angiotensin converting enzyme inhibition on renal function in patients with diabetic nephropathy." *British Medical Journal* 1986; 293: 471–474.

Bjorck, S., H. Mulec, S. A. Johnsen, G. Norden, M. Aurell. "Renal protective effect of enalapril in diabetic nephropathy." *British Medical Journal* 1992; 304: 339–343.

DeVenuto, G., G. Andreotti, M. Mattarei. "Prolonged treatment of essential hypertension and renal function: Comparison of captopril and beta-blockers considering microproteinuria values." *Current Therapeutic Research* 1985; 38(5): 718–728.

Elving, L. D., J. M. Wetzel, E. deNobel, et al. "Captopril reduces albuminuria probably through lowering of intraglomerular pressure, acute effects seen in patients with diabetic nephropathy." *Postgraduate Medical Journal* 1988; 63:34 (Abstract)

Holdaas, H., A. Hartman, M. G. Lien, L. Nilsen, J. Jervell, P. Fauchald, et al. "Contrasting effects of lisinopril and nifedipine on albuminuria and tubular transport function in insulin dependent diabetics with nephropathy." *Journal of Internal Medicine* 1991; 229: 163–170.

Hommel, E., H. Parving, E. Mathiesen, et al. "Effect of captopril on kidney function in insulin dependent diabetic patients with nephropathy." *British Medical Journal* 1986; 293: 467–70.

Hostetter, T. H., H. G. Rennek, B. M. Brenner. "The case for intrarenal hypertension in the initiation and progression of diabetic and other glomerulopathies." *American Journal of Medicine* 1982; 72: 375–380.

Kisch, E. S. "Captopril and proteinuria in diabetes mellitus." *Irish Journal of Medical Science* 1987; 23: 833–834.

Lewis, E. J., L. G. Hunsicker, R. P. Bain, R. D. Rohde. "The effect of angiotensin converting enzyme inhibition in diabetic nephropathy." *New England Journal of Medicine* 1993; 329: 1456–1462.

Loutzenhiser, R., M. Epstein. "Effects of calcium antagonists on renal hemodynamics." *American Journal of Physiology* 1985; 249: F619–629.

Mimran, A., A. Insua, J. Ribstein, et al. "Comparative effect of captopril and nifedipine in normotensive patients with incipient diabetic nephropathy." *Diabetes Care* 1988; 11: 850–853.

Parving, H. H., E. Hommel, M. D. Nielsen, et al. "Effect of captopril on blood pressure and kidney function in normotensive insulin dependent diabetics with nephropathy." *British Medical Journal* 1989; 299: 533–536.

Parving, H. H., E. Hommel, U. W. Smidt. "Protection of kidney function and decrease in albuminuria by captopril in insulin dependent diabetics and nephropathy." *British Medical Journal* 1988; 297: 1086–1091.

Romanelli, G., A. Giustina, A. Cimino, et al. "Short-term effect on microalbuminuria induced by exercise in normotensive diabetics." *British Medical Journal* 1989; 298: 284–288.

Slomowitz, L. A., R. Bergamo, M. Grosvenor, J. D. Kopple. "Enalapril reduces albumin excretion in diabetic patients with low levels of microalbuminuria." *American Journal of Nephrology* 1990; 10: 457–462.

Taguma, T., Y. Kitamoto, G. Futaki, et al. "Effect of captopril on heavy proteinuria in azotemic diabetics. *New England Journal of Medicine* 1985; 313: 1617–1620.

Valvo, E., V. Bedogna, P. Casagrande, et al. "Captopril in patients with type II diabetes and renal insufficiency: systemic and renal hemodynamic alterations." *American Journal of Medicine* 1988; 85: 344–348.

Viberti, G., C. E. Mogensen, L. C. Groop, J. F. Pauls. "Effect of captopril on progression to clinical proteinuria in patients with type I insulin-dependent diabetes mellitus and microalbuminuria." *Journal of the American Medical Association* 1994; 271: 275–279.

Index